ASHP's **Informatics PEARLS**

Michael Schlesselman, PharmD, FASHP

Director of IT Program Management
Lawrence & Memorial Hospital
New London, Connecticut

Bonnie Levin, PharmD, MBA

Corporate Assistant Vice President
Pharmacy Services
MedStar Health, White Oak Informatics Center
Silver Spring, Maryland

American Society of Health-System Pharmacists®
Bethesda, MD

Any correspondence regarding this publication should be sent to the publisher, American Society of Health-System Pharmacists, 7272 Wisconsin Avenue, Bethesda, MD 20814, attention: Special Publishing. The information presented herein reflects the opinions of the contributors and advisors. It should not be interpreted as an official policy of ASHP or as an endorsement of any product. The information contained in this program, and the companion workbook, are to be used as guidance.

Because of ongoing research and improvements in technology, the information and its applications contained in this text are constantly evolving and are subject to the professional judgment and interpretation of the practitioner due to the uniqueness of each pharmacy's role in compounding sterile preparations and the handling of hazardous drugs. The editors, contributors, and ASHP have made reasonable efforts to ensure the accuracy and appropriateness of the information presented in this document. However, any user of this information is advised that the editors, contributors, advisors, and ASHP are not responsible for the continued currency of the information, for any errors or omissions, and/or for any consequences arising from the use of the information in the document in any and all practice settings. Any reader of this document is cautioned that ASHP makes no representation, guarantee, or warranty, express or implied, as to the accuracy and appropriateness of the information contained in this document and will bear no responsibility or liability for the results or consequences of its use.

Director, Special Publishing: Jack Bruggeman

Acquiring Editor, Special Publishing: Hal Pollard

Senior Editorial Project Manager: Dana Battaglia

Page Design: Carol Barrer

Library of Congress Cataloging-in-Publication Data

ASHP's informatics pearls / [edited by] Bonnie Levin, Michael D. Schlesselman.
p. ; cm.
"A collection of Pearls from the 2007 Management Pearls session in Las Vegas"--Pref.
Includes bibliographical references and index.
ISBN 978-1-58528-201-2
1. Medical informatics. 2. Hospital pharmacies. I. Levin, Bonnie. II. Schlesselman, Michael D. III. American Society of Health-System Pharmacists. IV. ASHP Midyear Clinical Meeting (42nd : 2007 : Las Vegas, Nev.) V. Title: Informatics pearls. VI. Title: American Society of Health-System Pharmacists' informatics pearls.
[DNLM: 1. Clinical Pharmacy Information Systems--organization & administration--Congresses. 2. Drug Therapy--methods--Congresses. 3. Pharmacy--organization & administration--Congresses. QV 26.5 A827 2008]
R858.A867 2008
362.17'82--dc22
2008046806

ISBN: 978-1-58528-201-2

Contents

iii   Note From the Publisher

v   Preface

vii   Contributors

1   1— Trials, Tribulations, and Triumphs in the Selection of an Information System
Michael D. Schlesselman

7   2— Training on a New Healthcare System Technology
James L. Besier

15   3—Ten Tips for Improving Computer Provider Order Entry Implementation
Carol J. Hope

19   4— Going Paperless: The Creation of Online Forms
Ingrid K. Lewis

25   5— Medication Use Process Automation and System Integration
Mark H. Siska

33   6— Downtime Bytes!
Patrice S. Johnson

37   7— What Did You Do With My Medication?
Barbara L. Giacomelli

43   8—Barcodes: They're Not Just for Medication Administration Anymore
Lynn Ethridge

49   **9—Using Genealogy Data Linked to Hospital Records to Build a Unique Pharmacogenomic Research Resource**
Frederick S. Albright

57   **10—"If You Didn't Document It"…That's Old News**
Brent I. Fox and Georgia W. Fox

67   **11—The Catcher in the Rye: Learning from Community Pharmacists' Interventions on Electronic Prescriptions**
Terri L. Warholak and Michael T. Rupp

75   **12—Online Pharmacy Services Resource Center: A Concept URL Bound to Love**
Janet Jean Madsen

87   **Appendix A: ASHP Statement on the Pharmacist's Role in Informatics**

95   **Appendix B: Pharmacy Informatics Specialty Residency/Fellowship Programs**

99   **Index**

Note from the Publisher

The Pearls sessions at the ASHP Midyear Clinical Meeting (MCM) are some of the best attended sessions each year. With the publication of the "Pearls" series ASHP is attempting to capture the best of these presentations and add a depth of coverage and material that is not possible under the strict time constraints of the MCM pearls presentations. We hope you find this compilation worthwhile.

We encourage ASHP members to participate in the MCM Pearls presentations and for those that are selected to consider turning those presentations into chapters for the Pearls book series. For additional information on becoming a Pearls series author please contact me at jbruggeman@ashp.org

Preface

The American Society of Health-System Pharmacists has defined an "Informatic Byte" as an idea, concept, fact, or information that a pharmacist has found useful in their application of informatics and technology, but that "byte" may not be widely known, understood, published, or taught.

This is an exciting time for pharmacists who are interested in informatics because it is the newest specialty of pharmacy practice. Consequently, informatic bytes are the "new" kids on the block in the ASHP "pearl" sessions, as is the Section of Pharmacy Informatics and Technology. As technology and informatics become more engrained in the practice of pharmacy, the more important and valuable it is to have practitioners from all settings and practices share their collective knowledge through the "byte" sessions. The informatics bytes session are brief and to the point. But as you know, informatics and technology are anything but brief.

Here for the first time, we have attempted to capture in book form the expertise, value, and brevity that characterized these traditional ASHP presentations. Selected presenters have been asked to expand on their original presentations at the 2007 and 2008 ASHP Winter Meeting Informatic Bytes sessions to provide those who could not attend with the opportunity to access the information presented and to provide those who did attend more "depth" than was possible during the brief five minutes each speaker was afforded. So, whether you sat in on the session or not, there should be something useful for you in the pages that follow. And, perhaps these pearls will prompt you to consider submitting a pearl for the next Midyear Clinical Meeting, and we hope that these Bytes will help you improve your ability to use informatics to provide better and safer patient care.

Michael Schlesselman
Director of IT Program Management
Lawrence & Memorial Hospital
New London, Connecticut

Bonnie Levin
Corporate Assistant Vice President, Pharmacy Services
MedStar Health
Silver Spring, Maryland

Contributors

Frederick S. Albright, PhD
Director for CPCSS
College of Pharmacy
University of Utah
Salt Lake City, Utah
frederick.albright@pharm.utah.edu

James L. Besier, PhD, RPh, FASHP
BCMA Administrator, Pharmacy Residency Program Director
Health Alliance
Pharmacy Services
Cincinnati, Ohio
jim.besier@healthall.com

Lynn Ethridge, PharmD
Manager, Pharmacy Informatics
Greenville Hospital System
University Medical Center
Greenville, South Carolina

Brent I. Fox, PharmD, PhD
Assistant Professor
Auburn University
Harrison School of Pharmacy
Auburn, Alabama
foxbren@auburn.edu

Georgia W. Fox, PharmD, BCPS
Assistant Clinical Professor
Auburn University
Harrison School of Pharmacy
Auburn, Alabama
gfox@auburn.edu

Barbara L. Giacomelli, PharmD, MBA
Director of Pharmacy
Shore Memorial Hospital
Somers Point, New Jersey
bgiacomelli@shorememorial.org

Carol J. Hope, PharmD, MS
VA Ideas Center
VA Salt Lake City Healthcare System
Salt Lake City, Utah
carol.hope@utah.edu

Patrice S. Johnson, BS, PharmD
Clinical Pharmacist/Application Analyst
Children's National Medical Center
Washington, DC
PSJohnso@cnmc.org

Ingrid K. Lewis, PharmD, BCPS
Pharmacist
Clinical Application Services
The Children's Hospital
Aurora, Colorado
lewis.ingrid@tchden.org

Janet Jean Madsen, PharmD
Hospital Pharmacy Training & Knowledge Manager
Fairview Pharmacy Services
Minneapolis, Minnesota
jmadsen1@fairview.org

Michael T. Rupp, PhD, RPh
Professor of Pharmacy Administration
Midwestern University - Glendale
Glendale, Arizona
mtrupp@midwestern.edu

Mark H. Siska, RPh, MBA/TM
Mayo Clinic Rochester
Rochester, Minnesota
siska.mark@mayo.edu

Terri L. Warholak, PhD, RPh
Assistant Professor, Department of Pharmacy Practice & Science
College of Pharmacy-Pulido Center
Tucson, Arizona
warholak@pharmacy.arizona.edu

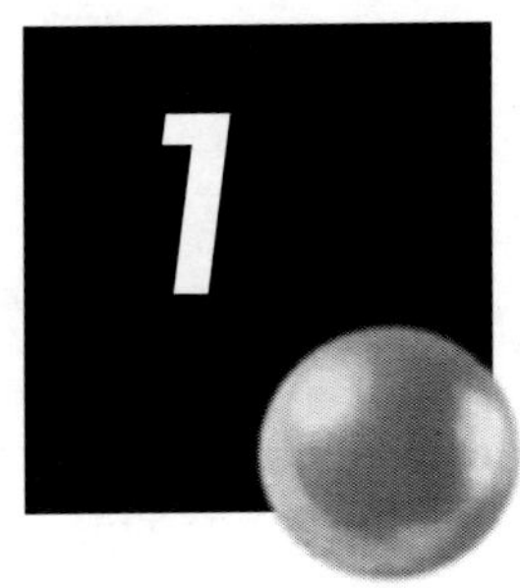

Trials, Tribulations, and Triumphs in the Selection of an Information System

Michael D. Schlesselman

Background and Introduction

Lawrence & Memorial (L&M) Hospital of New London, Connecticut had the desire and need to improve upon their existing information systems. L&M Hospital is a community, not-for-profit hospital in southeastern Connecticut. To ensure that L&M Hospital was using the best information system that best matched out needs, we embarked on a 1-year endeavor to find the best information technology (IT) solution for us. To obtain this goal, we wanted to ensure that we were objective as possible and eliminated as much bias as possible during the process. One of the most difficult aspects of selecting an IT solution is to separate fact from fiction, just as you would when selecting a medication for addition to or elimination from the formulary. Determining from marketing what is merely "smoke and mirrors" and what is actually available and installed can be a very daunting task, and any selection process that will involve many different departments and disciplines can become very emotional at times. Because of these factors, L&M Hospital created an objective, structured process to ensure that we stayed on target, eliminated bias, and found a means to minimize subjectivity.

Any endeavor to change an IT solution for the hospital needs the support of senior management starting at the President and Chief Executive Officer (CEO) level. L&M not only had this support, it also had the CEO's mandate that we obtain the best IT solution that fit our institution. With this mandate, the Chief Information Officer set a course to successfully meet this challenge. One of the first tasks was to create an IT steering committee made up of hospital leaders. The steering committee was made up of all directors leading clinical departments: the directors of finance, materials management, quality and risk management, and physician practice; managers of dietary, rehabilitation services, and case management; and senior management. This steering committee was supplemented with numerous IT department personnel who were involved throughout the process. There was also a parallel Physician IT Steering Committee made up of physicians from all areas of practice within the hospital. Many of the steps and processes used by the Hospital IT Steering Committee were also completed by the Physician IT Steering Committee.

Defining the Scope and Goals

One of the first tasks was to define the scope and goals for the selection process. The vendor we sought needed to have the products and services, results, financial obligations, technical aspects, and willingness to partner with us. As with any project, defining the scope at the beginning is critical to the success of the project. Defining the scope would allow the steering committees to stay on task and would help to prevent the vendors from taking us down a path we did not want to go down. The first and most important part of the scope was defining the products and services we were looking at. Our first criterion was to find a solution that offered an integrated clinical solution that would meet most, if not all, of our needs. This integrated clinical solution would also need to support L&M's desire to support the physician in the ambulatory setting. L&M felt that it was vitally important that physicians have an electronic solution in their offices, so when they came to the hospital they would not feel like they were having to learn a different way of doing their jobs. Another benefit is the data sharing that can occur if the physicians have electronic records in their office. The proposed solution would need to be user friendly and intuitive and allow for easy remote access. L&M is a very data-driven organization; the IT solution being sought would need to have reporting capabilities that would allow the organization to efficiently and effectively utilize the data in the clinical system. Integration of the system included supporting everything from the front end of scheduling to the back end of billing and everything in between. Ease of implementation was a critical piece of the puzzle. As with many organizations, people and resources are limited, and the solution we were seeking to implement needed to address these limitations.

L&M was looking for a company that had proven results and could clearly demonstrate the ability to create a solution that improved the delivery of care. As with a major purchase, there needed to be proof of a return on investment. Because implementation is so critical to the success of a project, we were looking for a vendor that had a proven track record in implementing their clinical solutions to the fullest extent of the product suite. We were not looking for a vendor that was really strong in one product and weak in another or had not implemented all of the modules. The vendor also needed to be able to engage the physicians in a positive manner, getting their participation and "buy in."

The financial obligation incurred with this project also needed to be supported by the organization, and, as such, the vendor needed to be able to present an affordable solution for both implementation and maintenance. L&M also looked at the additional staff needed to implement and maintain the system, knowing that the current IT department was not staffed for a major implementation. The IT department was looking for architecture that is easy to implement, support, and upgrade. A proven and effective customer service solution was also important in the selection process, and the KLAS® survey was used to help determine the vendors' response to customer service. L&M was also looking for a vendor that would align with our values and culture and would be willing to become a partner with L&M.

L&M further defined the clinical solutions that would be keys in the selection process. We provided a list of modules the vendors needed to support. With much emphasis on medication safety, the solution of choice must be able support a closed medication loop–system. This system includes supporting automation and information systems, such as automated dispensing cabinets, barcoded medication administration, IV smart pumps, automated total parenteral nutrition compounding and any other forward-looking technology. Tight integration between pharmacy, nursing, and computerized provider order entry was of utmost importance. Having these three products on the same platform with strong integration was a crucial criterion. There also needed to be support for our limited pediatric and neonatal population. Additionally, the solution needed to support lab outreach, physician portal, document imaging, single sign-on capability, psychiatric services, nurse data sets, mammography, automated charging, and surgery center capabilities.

The Elimination Process

Knock-out criteria were also developed. The knock-out criteria could eliminate a vendor at any point in the process. The knock-out criteria were centered on the company, products and services, technical aspects, cost, and references. If the company had the potential to be acquired or merged, was not a "fit" for our culture, or demonstrated unethical behavior or unstable financial status they would be eliminated from the process. If the products or services did not meet the breadth required, did not have ambulatory capabilities, lacked a comprehensive customer service program, or suggested an unacceptable implementation strategy, it would be eliminated from the process. The technical aspect of the product must meet the definition of being an integrated model and not an interfaced model. Interoperability was crucial in a successful partner. Technology employed by the vendor shouldn't be antiquated, complex, or difficult to maintain, and relative cost to competitors was also important. Finally, references from current clients, reputation of the vendor, and positive site visits were the final knock-out criteria that could eliminate a vendor from the process.

Consultant Assistance

This entire process was to be completed in less than 12 months. To help L&M Hospital complete this endeavor, a consultant company was used. The task of the consultant was to do as much of the background and legwork of accumulating supporting information as possible. The consultants provided market overviews and trends and, as such, provided a starting point for the hospital. The consultants also sat in on vendor presentation to help gather data and track any issues that were identified. The consultants we retained from the very beginning and had the responsibility of making sure we stayed true to the course we had set out. To help us stay on track they provided request-for-proposal (RFP) boilerplates so we did not have to spend precious time creating them. The departments then took the boilerplate RFP and customized it to their specifications. This RFP was also part of the final contract signed by the selected vendor and L&M. Once RFPs were sent out and received, the consultant was responsible for collating the results and summarizing them for the steering committee. The consultants also brought to L&M some guiding principles which helped the steering committee stay focused on the task at hand. Those principles were: "implementation begins with selection," "think process not department," "maintain and document objectivity," "use the data but trust your gut," and "make a commitment." These principles stressed for us that selection was not separate from implementation but is actually the first step toward successful implementation. They also stressed the need to think of the "big picture," not just the department; eliminate subjectivity as much as possible; rely not on the data but use your gut instinct to measure if the data were accurate; and, finally, make the commitment with full force and not second guess yourself.

Rank	Functionality
	Table 1.1. Top Ten Results Related to Functionality of Systems
1	Pharmacy
2	Order and result management
3	Barcode medication administration
4	Computerized provider order entry
5	Laboratory
6	Clinical decision support
7	Clinical documentation
8	Electronic medication administration record
9	Acute clinical data repository and electronic medical record
10	Radiology

The consultants were very valuable in helping to keep the process as objective as possible. They provided scoring cards for every interaction with vendors, from the first presentation to the final presentation. The score cards were designed to help make the process as objective as possible, which also allowed us to ensure that we were fair to all vendor presentations. The consultants also had the steering committee complete a paired comparison. The paired comparison is an exercise in which each system is compared to the others and ranked. For example, pharmacy was compared with lab and ranked on importance. There were 20 different systems compared. Each steering committee member completed the comparison three times. A different perspective was used each time (e.g., the member's current role, organizational needs, and patient safety). The top 10 results are summarized in Table 1.1. This process helped prioritize functionality for the steering committee as we viewed vendor demos and created demo scripts. The results of this exercise would be used if we felt we had equal vendors and needed a "tie breaker." It was encouraging to find that pharmacy applications ranked toward the top. This finding reinforced the value of the pharmacy in its role of patient safety.

The Selection Process

The first step in the process for L&M was to send out a request for information (RFI), casting a broad net to obtain information from all interested vendors. In this document we defined our scope. The RFI allowed us to determine which vendors could accommodate our scope and also allowed us to identify areas in which the vendor may need to be supplemented with another vendor. All vendors that responded to our RFI were invited to present to the steering committee. The vendors for the first presentation were asked to speak to how they could meet our scope and how they would address any shortcomings. We wanted to get to know the company, its philosophy, and its future direction and start to determine if we could partner with them. Vendors were asked to not give a demonstration at this time. As previously mentioned, a score card was used for these presentations, and, based on the score cards and information we collected from these presentations, we eliminated half of the vendors.

Those that made the cut were asked to present scripted demonstrations. Each area created scripts or orders for the specific applications that the vendor was to follow. We also created integrated demonstrations for the vendors to show complete functionality. The vendors were instructed to show only generally available products and note when they were showing versions that were not yet released. The goal of the scripted demonstrations was to prevent vendors from showing only their strengths. We realized that no vendor has the perfect solution, and part of the process was to see how the vendor addressed their weaknesses. From the scripted demonstrations we eliminated half of the vendors. Again each session was graded on score cards, which allowed us to keep the process objective. This phase of the process had the greatest input from staff members. Each application had a number of front-line staff members attend the scripted demonstrations. This process allowed the staff, the very workers who would be using the product, to evaluate and provide their comments. After this phase of the process we were down to two vendors.

With the remaining two vendors we did site visits and checked references. The site visits allowed us to determine if the vendor software packages worked as advertised in the "real world" as well as showing us a site that had the suite of products we were purchasing installed and live. We found that this was more challenging than we thought it would be. The vendors had difficulty finding sites that had the suite of products installed and using the products as advertised. Members of the hospital steering committee and some departmental managers went on the site visits. We tried to have the same people attend both vendors' sites to eliminate personal bias. The site visits created additional questions, which, in turn, required additional engagement of the vendors. As we got closer to making a final decision, we requested additional information and presentations from the vendors to answer lingering questions. This was also the stage in the process during which we openly and actively expressed concerns about holes in the functionality that we required the vendor to address to determine if we could live with these deficiencies. In most cases we felt we could work with the vendors' solutions and could fill gaps with niche products. We asked the two vendors to make one final summary presentation to wrap it up and make the final push to see which vendor we could ultimately work with.

The physicians worked in a process very similar to that of the hospital, and, as vendors were eliminated by the hospital, the physician steering committee made the same recommendations. In the early going, the physicians had a different ranking of the top two solutions but as time went along they arrived at the same recommendation as the hospital's. This was a win for everyone because we all agreed on the same solution. Thus, going forward there wouldn't be dissension because one group got their first choice.

Conclusion

In the end, we at L&M Hospital were able to settle on a vendor that had a similar philosophy as ours, had the solutions we were looking for, and had the vision we were looking for to grow with in the future. While we were able to complete this process in 12 months, the final contract signatures took much longer. We found that by applying objective tools to a subjective, emotional process we were able to make a decision that supported what we set out to do at the beginning, which was find a solution that met the needs of the organization and the physicians and would allow L&M to provide quality patient care.

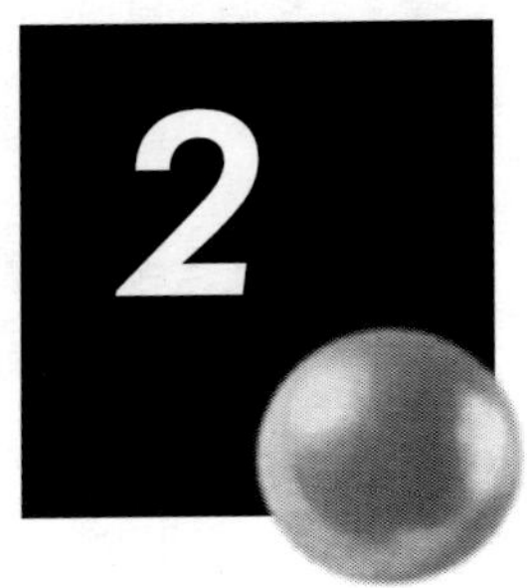

2 Training on a New Healthcare System Technology

James L. Besier

Background and Introduction

The utilization of technology has become integrated within the practice of pharmacy. In order to promote the focus on direct patient care activities and to reduce the emphasis on product orientation, increased implementation of technology and automation is imperative. With increased implementation into current pharmacy practice, workflow processes and practice models will be expected to change. This chapter will describe a strategy that was successfully used to educate and train healthcare professionals in the use of a newly implemented system-wide technology, review the theoretical framework used in the development of the educational and training strategy, and provide an example of the methods used in the education and training program.

In 2004, The Health Alliance of Greater Cincinnati, a group of six hospitals serving the greater Cincinnati region, embarked on a computerized provider order entry (CPOE) system implementation effort at two of its hospitals as part of the ongoing quality improvement efforts.[1] GE, formerly IDX, LastWord®, was the hospital information system (HIS) used at all facilities. It had been used for order management since 1998. The system was tailored and its processes redesigned for CPOE use. The pilot units were an orthopedic and neurosurgery unit at Christ Hospital (a community hospital with 555 beds) and a general surgery unit at the University Hospital (with 665 beds). The hospitals implemented CPOE on June 6, 2005 and September 7, 2005, respectively. At the community hospital, "universal" use was encouraged, whereas use was required at the university hospital. The two environments differed significantly in that the community hospital's patients had orders entered by staff physicians or physician assistants. The majority of orders were entered by house staff (residents and fellows) or medical students at the university hospital. In both settings, adopting CPOE was a significant undertaking that required extensive resources, process and cultural changes, and educational and training efforts.

Education and Training Program Development

The Health Alliance Department of Pharmacy Services had historically taken the responsibility for the education and training of all of its associates with respect to the implementation of new technology within the organization. Pharmacy trainers often used Health Alliance resources, such as corporate training and development materials and information systems and technology analysts, to assist in the development of education materials. Because all of the pharmacy associates that were selected to participate in CPOE training activities were adults with multiple years of experience in their respective departments, adult learning theory literature was reviewed prior to education and training program development. Malcolm Knowles developed andragogy, the process of engaging learners in the structure of their learning experiences, into a theory of adult education.[2] This theory has been characterized in the following way[3]:

- Adults are autonomous and self-directed.
- Adults have accumulated a foundation of life experiences and knowledge.
- Adults are goal oriented.
- Adults are relevancy oriented.
- Adults are pragmatic.
- Adults need to be shown respect.

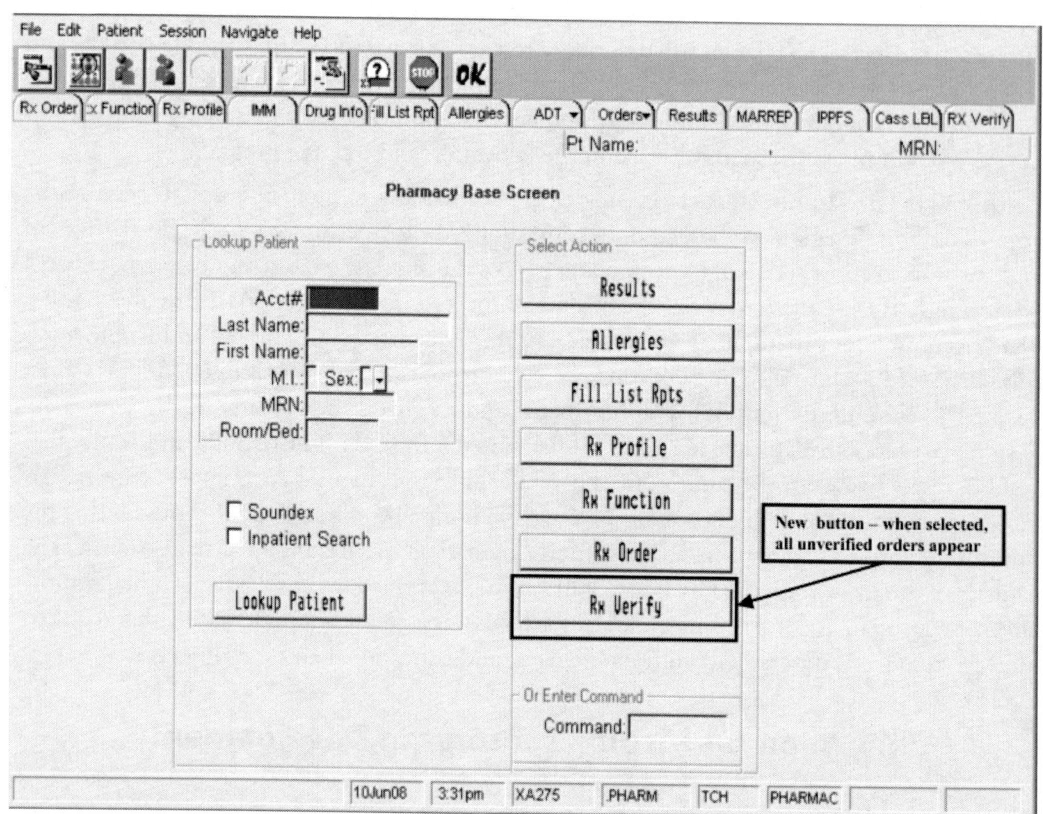

Figure 2.1. Pharmacy base screen.

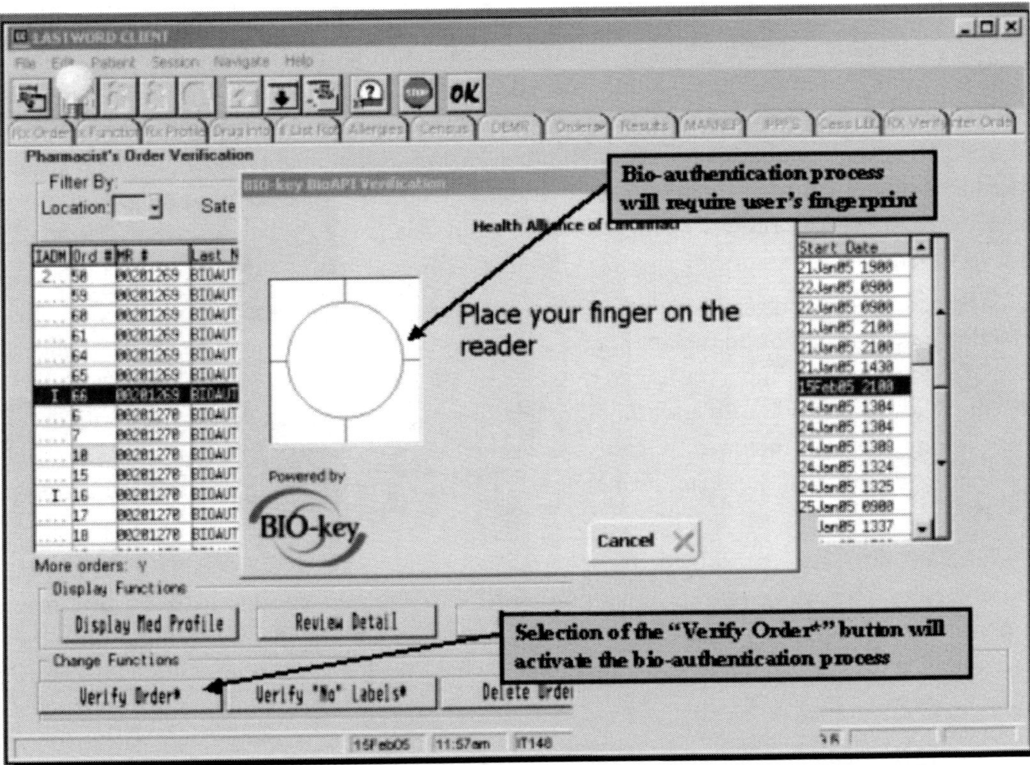

Figure 2.2. Bio-authentication screen.

More specifically, Knowles postulated that adult learners:

- Move from dependency to self-directedness.
- Draw upon their reservoirs of experience and learning.
- Are ready to learn when they assume new roles.
- Want to solve problems and apply new knowledge immediately.[2]

Covey has also explored the movement from dependence to interdependence or self-directedness.[4] In order to engage the participants in their training with the goal of optimizing the experience, the preceding characteristics were considered when developing the education and training materials.

In addition to adult learning theory literature, change model literature was also reviewed. A significant change in professional practice responsibilities would occur with the implementation of CPOE. Pharmacists would be progressively less involved in the medication order-entry process and more involved with order verification. Holland and Nimmo described the relationship of three basic components in their change model theory.[5-9] Two of the components, practice environment and learning resources, along with the application of Knowles' considerations, formed the basis of the pharmacy education and training materials and activities. Program sessions for trainees were 3 hours long and divided into distinct education and training components. Multiple groups of between 5 and 10 trainees attended sessions that were held approximately 3 weeks to 4 weeks before respective "go-live" events. Although the program was primarily designed for pharmacy associates, other organizational members could benefit from the education and training. Invitations to attend the sessions were extended to nonpharmacist members of the CPOE project team, care team, a physician, and consultants who were hired to help support associates during the two CPOE "go-live" events.

The education component of the program consisted of a slide presentation that formally provided new information to the attendees. A training manual that contained all of the slides presented in the session and a posting of the slides on the organization's intranet supplemented the education component. In addition, the slides were copied onto CD-ROMs for attendees' use. The information included, but was not limited to: screen shots from the new software application, definitional slides, and copies of new labels. Figures 2.1 and 2.2 provide examples of such slides.

Program organizers presumed that pharmacists would receive many calls from nurses and physicians requesting assistance with the order-entry process because it would be a new responsibility for the two groups. Thus, pharmacists would not only become familiar with the screen flow in their own application, but also those seen by other application users. Therefore,

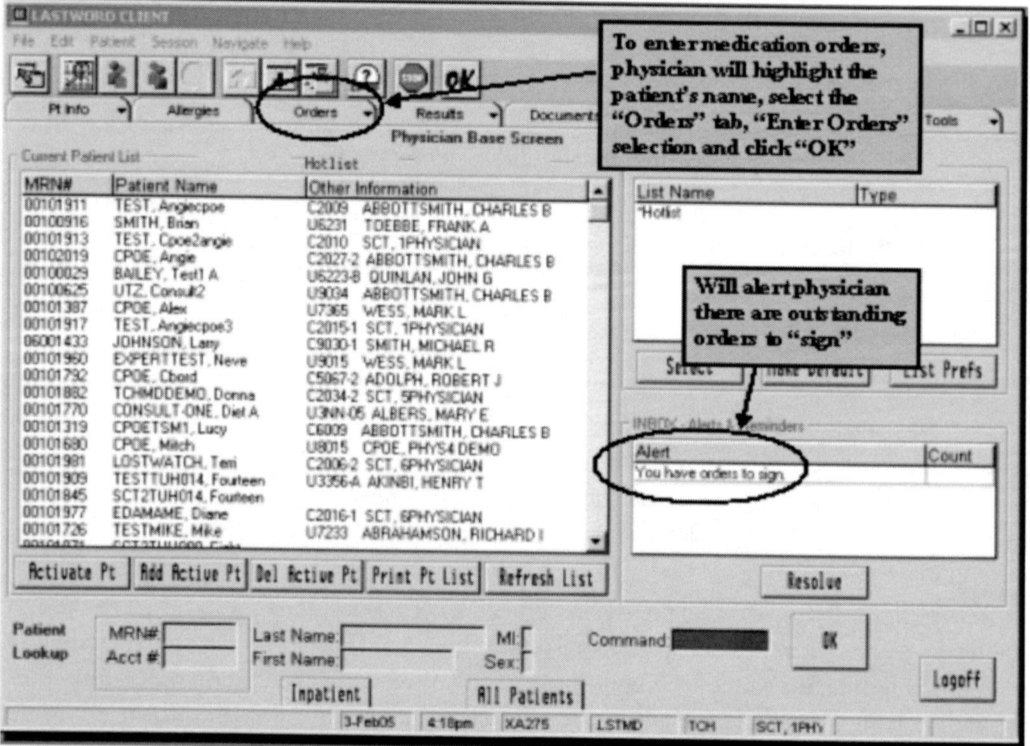

Figure 2.3. Physician base screen.

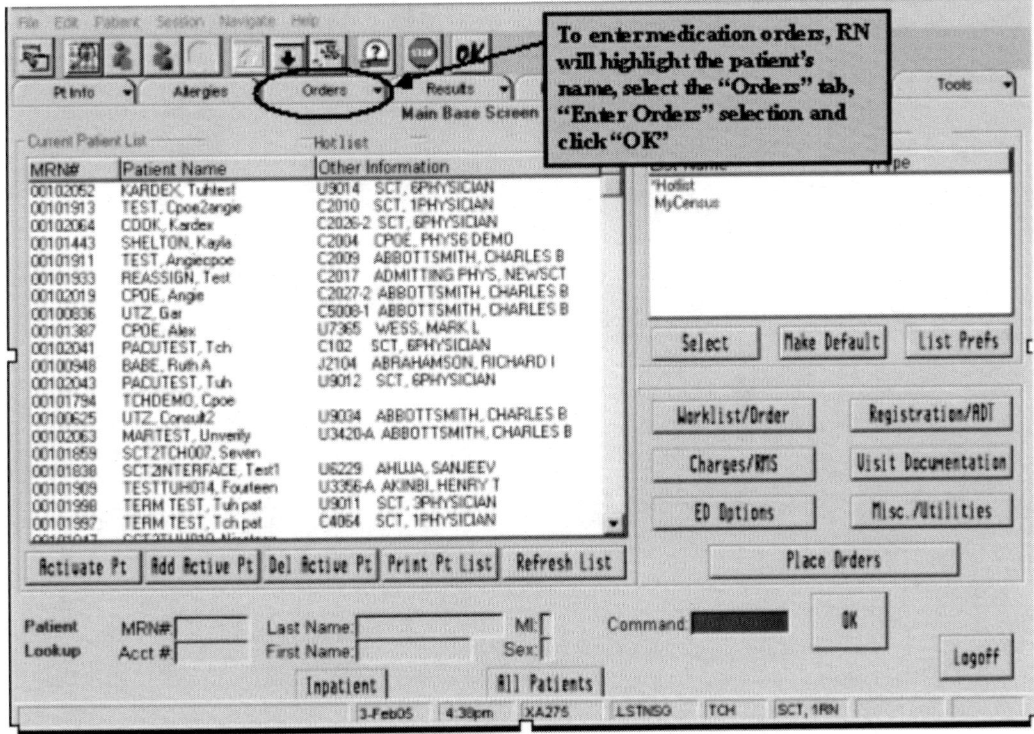

Figure 2.4. Nurse base screen.

physician and nurse application screen shots were also included in the pharmacy educational material (Figs. 2.3, 2.4).

In keeping with Knowles' contention that adult learners want to apply new knowledge immediately, the information systems and technology department was requested to develop virtual patient profiles on the HIS training pathway. The pharmacy trainer developed the patient profiles. The training pathway permitted trainees to practice new activities they had just learned without disrupting the real-life order entry process on actual in-house patients. The virtual patient profiles contained the following patient data: name, attending physician, account number, medical record number, room and bed location, allergies and intolerances, clinical notes and interventions, medications, dosages, routes, frequency, and start and stop dates (Fig. 2.5). At the beginning of each session, attendees were given a training manual and a sheet that provided data on a virtual patient. The data included a unique HIS training pathway user ID and password, patient name, account number, and medical record number. The user could simulate all of the activities presented in the education session in the training pathway with the exception of the application of fingerprint and proximity card positive identification (see Fig. 2.2).

Session attendees were provided approximately 1 hour to use the training pathway to practice activities and ask questions of the trainer. In addition, they were able to access the training pathway after the formal session to gain additional experience with the new application. Toward the conclusion of the 3-hour session, attendees were requested to complete two different documents: a five-question Pharmacy CPOE Training Evaluation and a 13-question Pharmacy CPOE

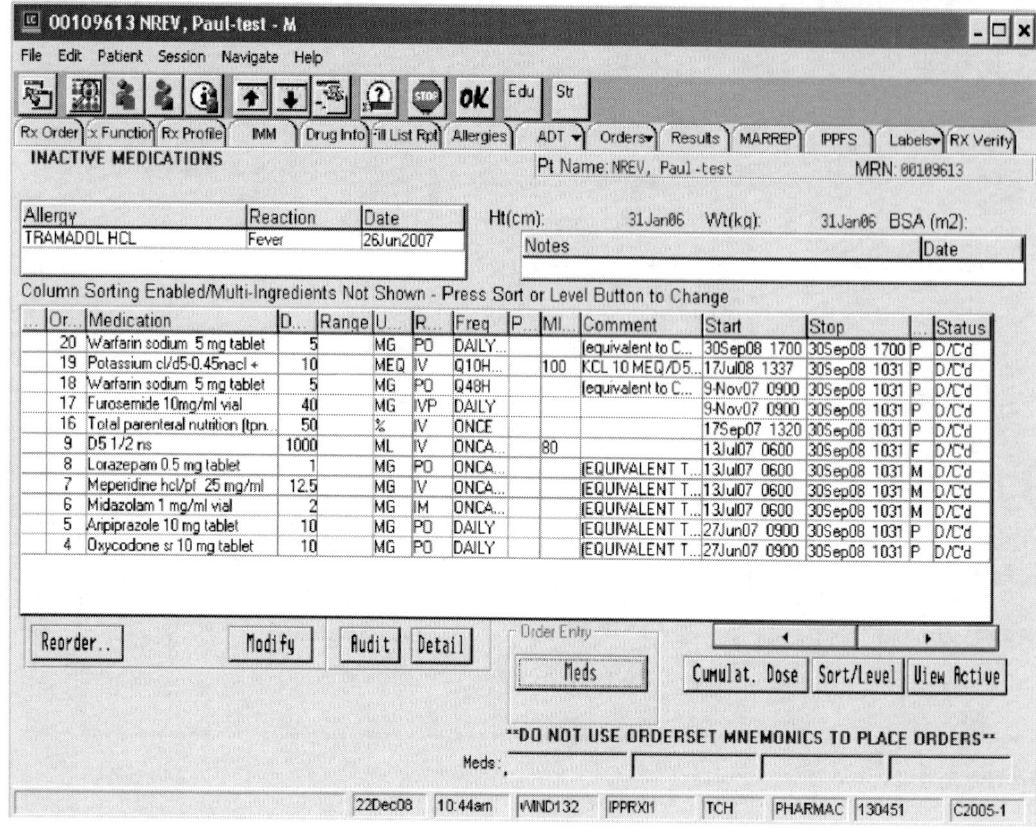

Figure 2.5. Active medication screen.

Assessment. The training evaluation provided insight with respect to the attendee's assessment of the trainer's ability and organization, the usefulness of the handouts and training pathway, and the degree to which the program's objectives were achieved. The CPOE assessment document was a paper and pencil test of the attendee's comprehension of the information presented in the session. Based on the analysis of scores from both sets of documents, the education and training sessions were successful in providing information to the attendees. Overall, scores of 4.4 out of 5.0 were achieved on the training evaluation, and attendees achieved a mean score of 94% on the CPOE assessment.

Conclusion

An analysis of the scores from both documents, along with discussions with attendees after the conclusion of the education and training sessions, provided evidence that the program materials and presentations had been successful in preparing pharmacy associates to assume new roles and responsibilities with respect to the CPOE initiative. Understanding that adult learners approach the educational process somewhat differently than children do and providing the opportunity to practice new learning immediately may have enhanced the positive outcomes associated with the education and training sessions developed for the implementation of this new technology.

References

1. Wess ML. Effect of a computerized provider order entry (CPOE) system on medication orders at a community hospital and university hospital. Paper presented at: American Medical Informatics Association Annual Symposium; November 13, 2007; Chicago, IL.
2. Knowles MS. *The Modern Practice of Adult Education: From Pedagogy to Andragogy.* Revised ed. Cambridge Book Company; 1988.
3. Lieb S. Principles of adult learning. Available at: http://honolulu.hawaii.edu/intranet/ committees/FacDevCom/guidebk/teachtip/adults-2.htm. Accessed February 15, 2005.
4. Covey SR. *The Seven Habits of Highly Effective People.* New York: Simon & Schuster; 1989.
5. Holland RW, Nimmo CW. Transitions, part 1: beyond pharmaceutical care. *Am J Hosp Pharm* 1999;56:1758-1764.
6. Holland RW, Nimmo CW. Transitions in pharmacy practice, part 2: who does what and why. *Am J Hosp Pharm* 1999;56:1981-1987.
7. Holland RW, Nimmo CW. Transitions in pharmacy practice, part 3: effecting change—the three-ring circus. *Am J Hosp Pharm* 1999;56:2235-2241.
8. Holland RW, Nimmo CW. Transitions in pharmacy practice, part 4: can a leopard change its spots? *Am J Hosp Pharm* 1999;56:2458-2462.
9. Holland RW, Nimmo CW. Transitions in pharmacy practice, part 5: walking the tightrope of change. *Am J Hosp Pharm* 2000;57:64-72.

Ten Tips for Improving Computer Provider Order Entry Implementation

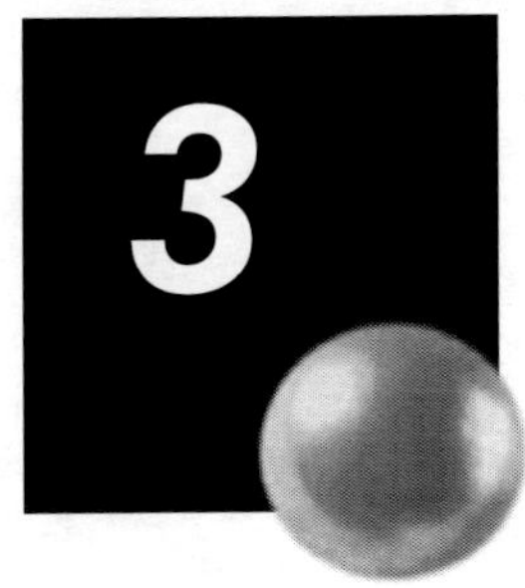

Carol J. Hope

Background and Introduction

Implementation of computerized provider order entry (CPOE) may be difficult, especially for someone not acquainted with the process. It is a time of socio-technological change, which can be very stressful for many people. When change is coupled with methods used for patient care, emotions may run high. Everyone is invested in maintaining good patient care, and many have strong feelings about how patient care is carried out. When CPOE is introduced, it must be customized not only to the manner of drug use, but also to the site's culture.

CPOE can be installed with either good or bad results. It is not automatically a "win-win" situation. Briefly, one of the benefits of CPOE is that it eliminates legibility problems; on the other hand, it introduces mistakes from incorrect key strokes or misplaced clicks. Juxtaposition becomes a problem. CPOE can also help with turn-around times to get medication to a patient faster. On the other hand, it makes it easy to leave an order in limbo, waiting to be cosigned.

The Steps

1. **Turning oranges into apples.** Watch for changes in the type of medication errors that occur. It's as if someone has changed oranges into apples. The "oranges," or old types of mistakes, are familiar to pharmacists, who are accustomed to looking for those particular types of mistakes, and they catch most of them. "Apples," or new types of mistakes, in many ways, are easier to correct and soon they will become as familiar as the old errors. The point is to watch for new types of mistakes and know they are coming.

2. **Problems may still be problems.** Some existing problems are likely to persist. Track your system's problem drugs. Current problems with sliding-scale insulin doses will probably continue, for example. The extra starting dose will still be needed when the medication is ordered for every morning and it is 3 PM already. If a drug will require different amounts of diluents for the amount of drug ordered, such as IgG, problems with it will probably continue even with the implementation of CPOE. New methods need to be carefully considered for these issues. Drugs that present problems in your pharmacy need

to be reviewed carefully in the new CPOE system.

3. Keep positives positive. Just like you track your old problems, the items that work well in the old system need to be monitored until you see how they work in the new system. If the process does not work, develop a new alternative. Know how to handle routine orders before implementation day. It is helpful to standardize order entry screens. Just like in the paper world, order sets may simplify the workload. Use well-thought-out maximum and minimum dosages. A quality decision support system can be very helpful.

4. Be proactive. In the very beginning when CPOE is being considered, it is helpful to get clinical pharmacists from the appropriate specialties, along with pharmacy system analysts, as members of the initial development and implementation committees. A pharmacist's viewpoint of what is needed to fill an order is much different than the viewpoint of a provider or nurse. The initial drug orders can be set up appropriately to avoid changing them later. A drug order can also be more difficult to change after others have already created its format. Orders will fit into a few set patterns with some additional outliers. Attending the early meetings can stop many problems that would otherwise occur on implementation day.

5. Be prepared. An ounce of prevention is worth a pound of afterthought. One of the most important items for CPOE implementation is to be prepared. Some of the pharmacists need to be trained as "super users" who know how to correct problems—as well as how to enter drugs. These super users can help the other pharmacists if someone from pharmacy informatics is not immediately available. Because you know up front that it will take longer to process orders during the conversion to CPOE, have additional staff on each shift. If the workload per pharmacist is reduced, the stress on any one person is not as great. Also, encourage other personnel who will use the system to be trained, including the providers when possible.

6. Measuring success is in the details. After implementation, the indicators that measure the results need to be carefully evaluated. For example, concluding that the providers entered 95% of their own orders may sound good, but when you determine that 50% of the orders have to be reentered by pharmacists, the results are less rosy.

7. A watched pot never boils. Stay out of trouble by handling problems immediately. Pharmacy system analysts need to be available 24 hours a day and on the floors as much as possible during the first 2 weeks of start-up, which will allow them to see the problems occur and catch them on the fly. With fewer corrections to be made and less people involved, a one-time problem is easier to handle than a problem that has occurred multiple times. Commonly, system analysts are available for the first 24 hours but additional problems will occur later. By staying in phone contact and attending shift change meetings, problems can be stopped in the early stages. The system analysts need to carefully listen to the staff and have the staff explain examples of the problems. After implementation, changes will still be required, but the pace will slow down.

8. The pharmacist's role continues. Some staff may think that they can just click on a medication to order it, and the medication is automatically dispensed by a Pyxis or similar machine. Somehow, the work of the pharmacist is forgotten. For most drugs, the pharmacist still needs to review the order before releasing it to be dispensed. The pharmacist's training and knowledge continue to be necessary; a pharmacist can prevent errors and save lives. Although medication turnaround may decrease with CPOE, pharmacy must still be part of the medication delivery process. Let staff know ahead of time that CPOE does not mean a fully automated process. If they have a realistic view of what CPOE can do, they are more likely to accept it.

9. **Take your donepezil.** Always remember paper order entry. When there is a power failure or the computer goes down, the drugs still have to be given to the patients. Document the procedures currently used so that they can be recalled when needed. Also, establish recovery procedure for post-downtimes.

10. **Sprinkle liberally with food.** Provide free food when initially implementing CPOE. It keeps everyone in good spirits. If the day is getting really bad and nothing seems to lift the team's mood, pass out candy. Chocolate can do wonders.

Conclusion

Know what your CPOE system can do for you and what the pharmacist's role continues to be. Be willing to adapt to the new system and soon you will not want to give up CPOE.

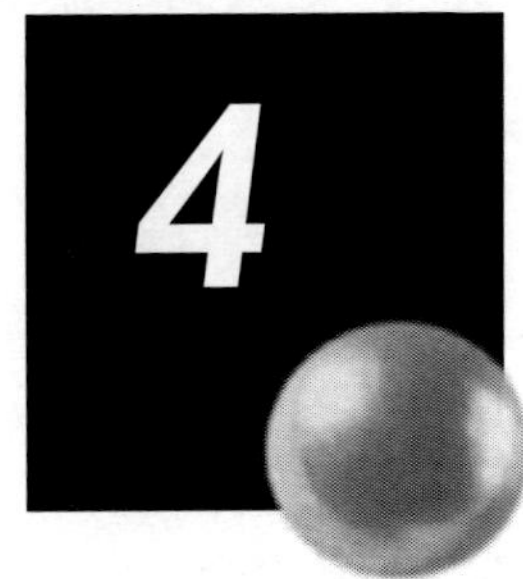

Going Paperless: The Creation of Online Forms

Ingrid K. Lewis

Background and Introduction

Switching from paper to online forms can streamline and improve workflow in the pharmacy. Designing and deploying an online pharmacy form can present unique challenges, however. Pharmacy forms need to fit the pharmacy workflow and provide solutions to the mounds of documentation required. Included in this chapter are pearls on designing and implementing a form.

Common online forms used by pharmacy facilities include the Adverse Drug Reaction, Medication Error, Medication Area Inspection, Intervention, Drug Information, Non-Formulary Request, and Batch Compounding Forms. The Joint Commission requirement for this information collection and retrieval has propelled their use. To comply with these requirements, many facilities use in-house forms available on their own Intranet. Other sites have opted to use forms from vendors with predesigned or customizable forms. Vendors include Pendragon, Pharmacy OneSource, and MedKeeper (sold through Gold Standard, Inc.).

Designing the Online Form

Administrators may be skeptical about the use of online forms and their acceptance by the pharmacy staff. Creating a straightforward, all-inclusive, and easy-to-complete form is the key. Once the type of form to be created is decided, work closely with your information technology department or vendor, pharmacists, and other users to get the most comprehensive form for your facility. Use the following list to add the best elements to your form.

1. **Select the best data entry field type for faster and easier documentation.** Drop-down boxes, text boxes, and radio buttons can all be used to enhance the form.[1] Drop-down boxes are used when selecting one item from a list (Fig. 4.1). They are ideal for static lists, such as locations, or for creating item categories such as a field for entering "Type of Adverse Drug Event." A drop-down list may also be ideal for an intervention list.

Adverse Drug Reactions

Patient Information

Patient Name: ________ Admit Date: ________

Room: ________ Discharge Date: ________

Med Record: ________ Prescribing MD: ________

Age: ________ Department: Pharmacy

Sex: ○ Male ○ Female Diagnosis: ________

Entered by: ________ Title ________

Reaction

Suspected Reaction: Allergic

Was the ADR the reason for admission? ○ Yes ○ No

Was Pt. on drug prior to admission? ○ Yes ○ No

Was ADR preventable? ○ Yes ○ No

Describe reaction: ________

Suspected Medications

Date of Reaction: 2008-03-18 All dates in yyyy-mm-dd format

Medication	Dose, Route, Interval	Start of Therapy	End of Therapy

Laboratory Values

Date	Labs	Date	Labs

Patient Outcome (check all that apply)

☐ Pt expired due to ADR ☐ FDA aware of ADR ☐ Pt educated

☐ ADR was life threatening ☐ MD aware of ADR ☐ MD educated

☐ ADR caused disability ☐ Medication held

☐ Pt required hospitalization ☐ Medication discontinued

☐ Hospitalization prolonged

☐ Pt expired NOT due to ADR

Reviewed By

Figure 4.1. Adverse drug event form with drop-downs, multi-select boxes, and calendar.

Instead of allowing each pharmacist to create his or her own intervention name, require selection from a list. This standardization keeps the data uniform and allows for groupings of categories when consolidating the report. Check boxes can be used when selecting multiple items from a list such as tracking outcomes from an adverse drug event ([ADR]i.e., hospitalization was prolonged, ADR caused disability, or ADR was life-threatening). Also, adding a calendar function allows the user to quickly pick a date.

2. **Design the form to follow the workflow.** Do not complicate the form by presenting it in an illogical sequence (i.e., one that does not follow the workflow). Your form can outline the steps involved in the process and sequence them so that the task may be completed in an orderly fashion. One example is a Non-Formulary Request Form on which progress on the acquisition of a drug can be tracked. The University of Colorado Hospitals recently made their Non-Formulary Request Form available to online users.[2] Their form consists of three sections. First, there is a section for the requestor to complete that triggers an approval mechanism. Once the request is approved, the next section delineates the process for drug acquisition. Finally, the last section is completed by the storeroom personnel who estimate the arrival date. The requestor can easily see the progress of the order.

3. Make old data easily retrievable. Another advantage of online forms includes the easy access to historical information. Query pages allow for searching of historical forms by date or other data field and for quick retrieval of previously completed forms. Alternatively, completed forms can be stored in folders grouped by date or type for easy referral back to the data. Retrieval of old forms is useful for almost all types of forms, especially with the new emphasis on regulation USP <797> batch and compounding information.[3]

4. Make the reports impressive. Collecting data in the proper format allows for the creation of colorful and notable reports summarizing the information collected (Fig. 4.2). By restricting the user to preselected lists, your data should be logically grouped and formatted. One strategy to designing a form may be to work backward and create the report to be presented to your administrator. Creating the data collection form after the report will ensure that all data points are included. Reports can be generated from an Excel spreadsheet or with commercial programs such as JFreeChart with a free software library for creating charts.[4]

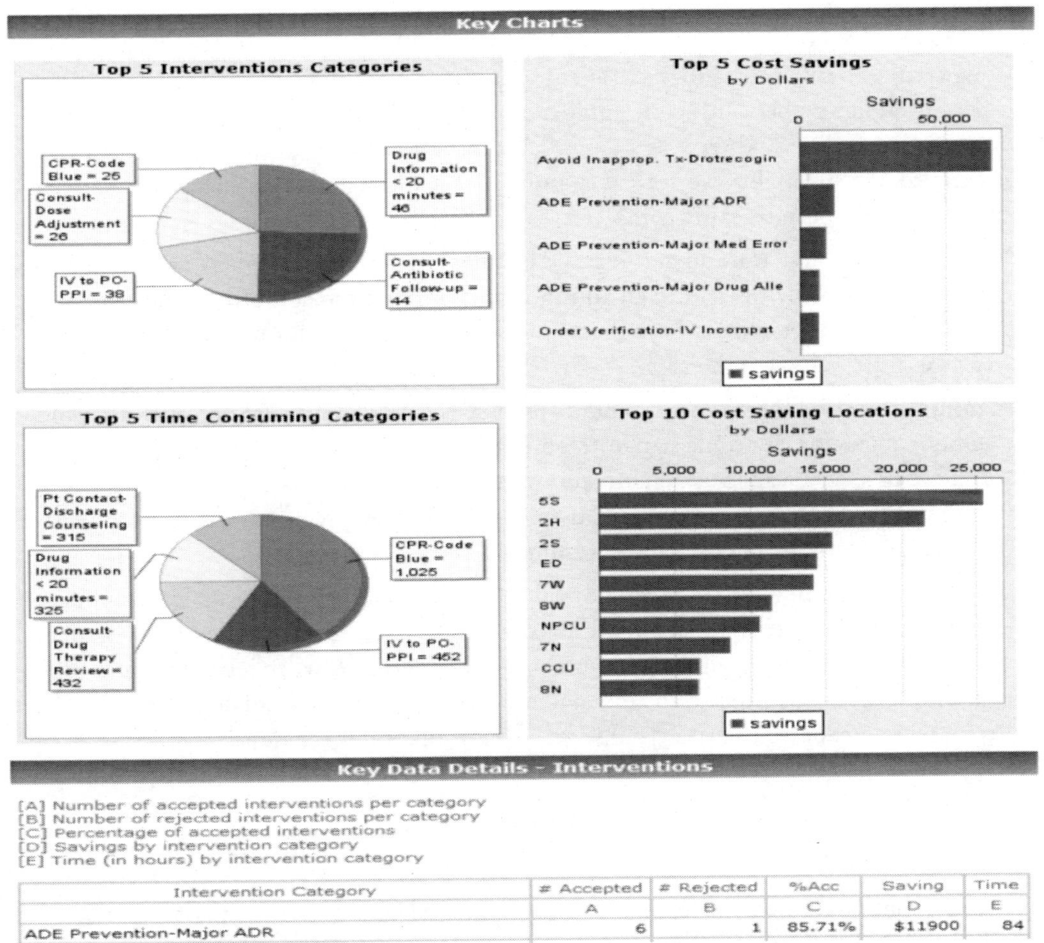

Intervention Category	# Accepted	# Rejected	%Acc	Saving	Time
	A	B	C	D	E
ADE Prevention-Major ADR	6	1	85.71%	$11900	84

Figure 4.2. Reports with multiple tables and graphs.

5. Plan for multiple drafts of the form. Before allowing access to all users, conduct a trial run with a few users and ask for feedback. Are all of the necessary fields available? Are all of the questions clearly presented? Is the information requested in a logical order? Based on the feedback, consider making changes to the form before allowing access to all users. Data may be lost if changes are made later.

Limitation of Online Forms . . . Possible Solutions

Don't be discouraged if your form cannot satisfy all of the requirements requested by the staff. Begin with a simple form and adapt it as new technologies become available. Here are a few stumbling blocks that can decrease a form's utility.

1. Too many comment fields. Users may complain that not enough comment fields are available throughout the form. While generous use of comment fields may make the form seem more complete, it may also make the form lengthy and unwieldy, especially on a personal digital assistant (PDA). Try adding one comment field after several questions and program it to expand as more information is added.

2. Difficult to collect information on a PDA. Typing long strings of information on a PDA can be tedious and time consuming (unless you have the experience of a phone-texting teen). Allow the user to make a "stub" on the PDA with fields such as patient name, identification number, and room number typed into the appropriate form to begin entry.[5] The stub should serve as a reminder to complete the form later. Once the PDA is synced, the stub will serve as the beginning of the form, and other fields, including any large text fields, can be easily completed using the computer keyboard.

3. Routing the form. Create an automatic e-mailing function so that when a form is completed, an e-mail alert is sent to an administrator or nurse for sign-off. In these cases, nurses or other users should have the appropriate access to the form and be able to either *view* or *make changes* to the form.

4. Signing the online form. Many vendors provide electronic signature options. To avoid additional fees for electronic signatures, one solution is to provide a special password to those users who can check off an approval box on the form. The form can be programmed so that only these "special" users may check the box. Allowing some type of electronic approval will save paper and time.

5. Too much data entry. HL7-integration allows for the sharing of information from different computer systems. Data fields such as patient name, room numbers, and patient identifiers may be auto-populated into a form. For example, when a patient name is selected from a look-up box, the remainder of the data is auto-populated. Auto-population, therefore, prevents extra typing and duplication of information.

Conclusion

The use of online forms is increasing. Good form design is crucial to the acceptance and use of the form. Having a well-organized and easy-to-complete form that is retrievable and provides impressive reporting should make the form more readily accepted. Adding advanced functionality, such as expanding comment fields, PDA stub reminders, e-mail alerts, electronic signatures or approval, and HL7-integration may make the electronic form preferred over the paper form.

References

1. The University of Melbourne Information Services. Web development centre. Available at: http://www.unimelb.edu.au/webcentre/tools/styleguide/forms.html. Accessed March 18, 2008.
2. Ferretti K [phone]. Denver, CO: University of Colorado Hospital; September 30, 2007.
3. United States Pharmacopeia, Inc. Chapter <797>: Pharmaceutical compounding—sterile preparations. Available at: http://www.usp.org/pdf/EN/USPNF/generalChapter797.pdf. Accessed March 18, 2008.
4. JFreeChart. Products and services. Available at: http://www.object-refinery.com/jfreechart/. Accessed March 18, 2008.
5. Fox BI, Felkey BG, Berger BA, et al. Use of personal digital assistants for documentation of pharmacists' intervention: a literature review. *Am J Health-Syst Pharm* 2007;64:1516-1525.

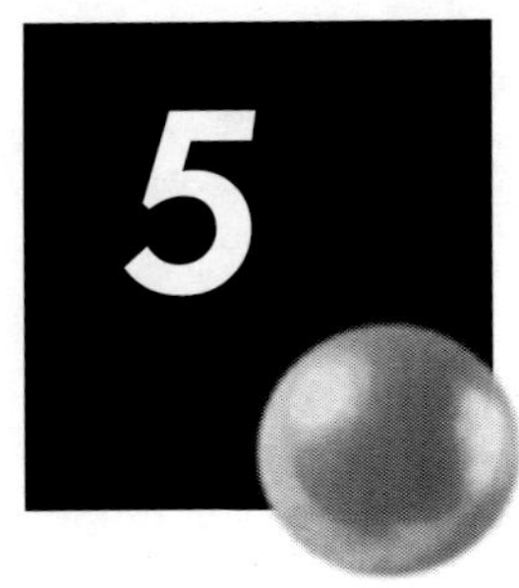

Medication Use Process Automation and System Integration

Mark H. Siska

Background and Introduction

In 2000, The Institute of Medicine (IOM) Report titled, "To Err is Human: Building a Safer Health System," documented that medication errors represents the largest single cause of medical errors in the hospital, accounting for more than 7,000 deaths annually. The report made it clear that to improve medication safety, healthcare organizations must "implement proven medication safety practices" to reduce reliance on memory; standardize terminology; utilize constraints, forcing functions, protocols, and checklists; and minimize data handoffs. The report made reference to several emerging technologies and systems that may be used to effectively reduce medical errors, particularly in hospital settings.[1]

IOM's second report, "Crossing the Quality Chasm: A New Health System for the 21st Century," was more emphatic about the use of information technology in the redesign of health care systems to improve quality and reduce errors. The report called for automation of patient-specific clinical information within the context of an electronic health record and integrated with computerized physician order entry (CPOE) systems, drug distribution, and administration systems.[2] These systems could transmit electronic orders seamlessly to downstream performing departments and, coupled with real-time patient-specific clinical information and decision support, could potentially reduce errors and improve overall patient safety. The human as well as financial cost of medication errors and recommended solutions for improvement prompted the healthcare industry, large healthcare purchasers, and state and federal governments to adopt and implement health information technology (IT) solutions to minimize medication-related errors. The suggested improvements meant that organizations would need to re-engineer existing error-prone medication-use processes by introducing additional systems to support the end-to-end management and communication of medications across the continuum of care. It has been over 8 years since the IOM report was published, suggesting the use of a variety of systems to address some of the deficiencies and safety concerns in the medication use process. Additional systems have been suggested to further integrate a complex set of processes and corresponding functions to "close the loop" and achieve the "ideal medication-use cycle." Many healthcare organizations have made significant efforts to implement electronic systems to assist with reducing medication errors by targeting specific

Hospital Information
(Answer all that apply)

System Type

Bed Size

Community Hospital

Owner/Control

Teaching Status

Location

Pharmacy Practice Model
What best describes the current pharmacy practice model in your facility?
  *Clinical refers to a proactive practice with or without formalized programs
  *Traditional refers to a reactive practice primarily focusing on distribution

Unit based (decentral) clinical
Unit based (decentral) traditional
Central based clinical
Central based traditional
Central based clinical and traditional
Unit (decentral) and central based clinical and traditional
Other

If other, please describe:

What best describes your pharmacy's primary mode of dispensing scheduled (batchfill) medications? (Select all that apply)

☐ Manual Cart Fill

☐ Automated Cart Fill

☐ Automated Dispensing Cabinets

☐ Other (Please Describe)

Please choose what best describes the status of an Electronic Medical Record in your organization.

Figure 5.1. Medication-use system deployment survey.

phases of the medication-use process. A recent American Society of Health System Pharmacist national survey of pharmacy practice in hospital settings indicates a growing trend toward the implementation of safer medication distribution and administration systems.[3] The adoption of automated dispensing cabinets linked to patients' medication profiles, barcode assisted medication administration (BCMA), electronic medication administration records, smart infusion pumps, and CPOE systems have all increased significantly over the past several years. Despite the evidence supporting the continued deployment of medication management systems, it's difficult to assess the current degree of medication management system integration. Healthcare IT surveys and questionnaires clearly indicate medication management system deployment; however, evidence examining current trends related to system integration or interoperability are absent from the literature.

System and Automation Integration and Interoperability Survey

To determine current trends in medication-use system deployment, a survey was developed to determine not only the number of medication management supporting technologies and automation currently deployed but also the number of integration and interoperability opportunities realized (Fig. 5.1).

Medication Management Supporting Systems

Select all the medication use process supporting systems implemented (or soon to be implemented) within your organization.

- ☑ Medication Order Management Systems
- ☑ Pharmacy Information Management Systems
- ☑ Automated Workflow Management & Inventory Management Systems
- ☑ Unit Dose and Bar Code Packaging Systems
- ☐ Automated Sterile Compounding Devices
- ☐ Automated Medication Cart Fill or Envelope Fill Systems
- ☐ CPOE
- ☐ Intelligent Infusion Pumps
- ☐ Bedside Medication Verification/EMAR
- ☐ Clinical Intervention Documentation System
- ☐ Electronic Medical Record
- ☐ Clinical Decision Support Systems
- ☐ Automated Dispensing Cabinets

Figure 5.2. Medication management support automation and systems.

Active primary and secondary members of the American Society of Health System Pharmacist's Section of Informatics and Technology representing a wide variety of health systems across the United States were surveyed by e-mail. The survey focused on 13 distinct medication management supporting automation and systems currently deployed in healthcare organizations (Fig. 5.2).

Members were polled to select the medication-use process supporting systems implemented or soon to be implemented within their organizations. Assuming complete integration across the entire medication-use process as the ideal, respondents choosing multiple systems or automa-

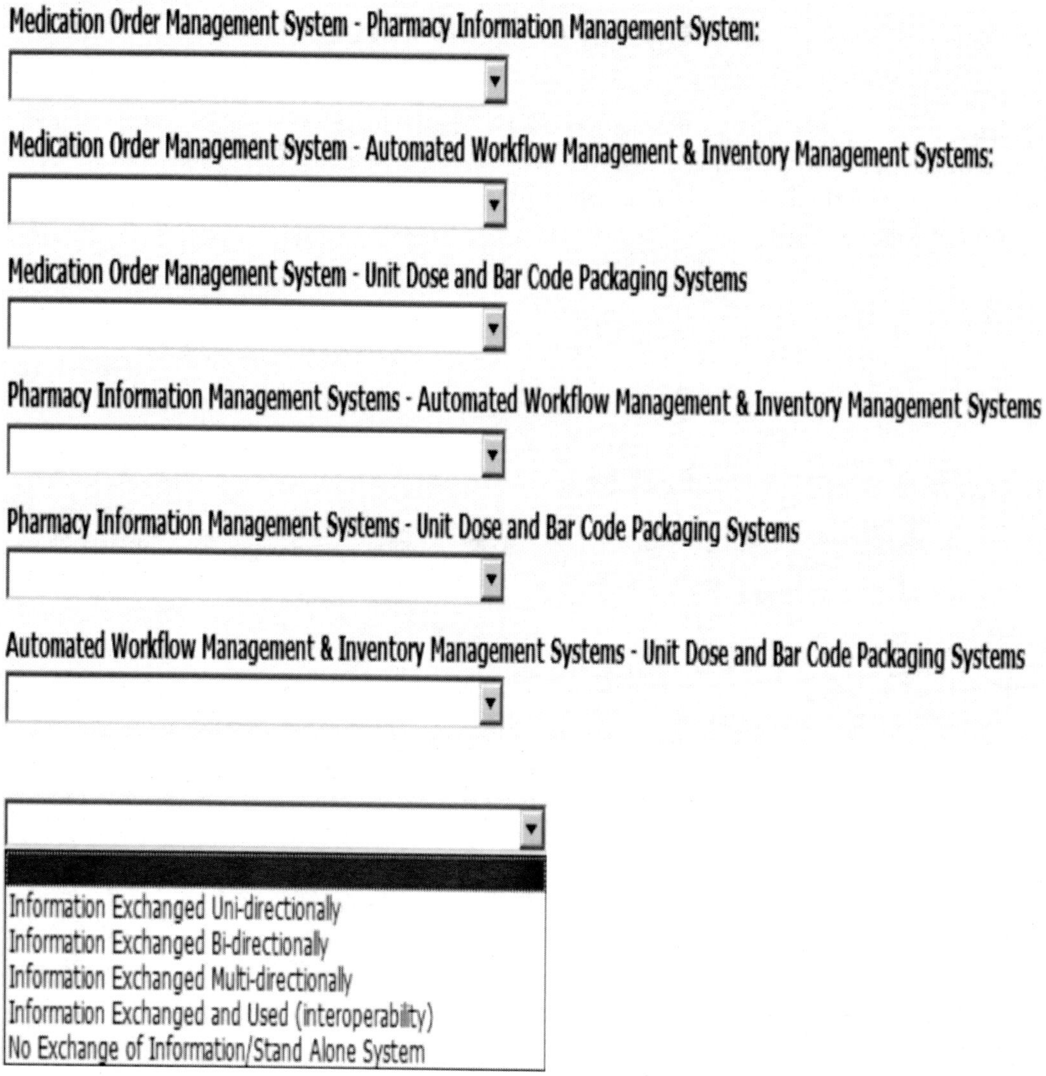

Medication Order Management System - Pharmacy Information Management System:
Medication Order Management System - Automated Workflow Management & Inventory Management Systems:
Medication Order Management System - Unit Dose and Bar Code Packaging Systems
Pharmacy Information Management Systems - Automated Workflow Management & Inventory Management Systems
Pharmacy Information Management Systems - Unit Dose and Bar Code Packaging Systems
Automated Workflow Management & Inventory Management Systems - Unit Dose and Bar Code Packaging Systems

Information Exchanged Uni-directionally
Information Exchanged Bi-directionally
Information Exchanged Multi-directionally
Information Exchanged and Used (interoperability)
No Exchange of Information/Stand Alone System

Figure 5.3. Degree of system integration and interoperability in survey.

tions were asked to indicate the degree of system integration and interoperability as described in Figure 5.3. Each pair of systems selected was considered an opportunity for integration or interoperability.

Survey Results

Fifty-one surveys were completed with respondents indicating an average of 6 to 7 distinct medication management supporting systems implemented within their organization. There were 1,054 potential opportunities identified by respondents for systems implemented to share information with other medication management supporting systems and automations. Responding organizations took advantage of integration in 50% of all potential opportunities, indicating no exchange of information taking place between systems. Forty percent of the opportunities were realized with some level of exchange and 10% of the opportunities were fully realized through interoperability.

Ninety percent of health systems polled had automated the medication management distribution process, indicating that they had implemented both a pharmacy information management system (PIMS) and automated dispensing device, including cabinets or robotics with 70% of respondents reporting some level of exchange or integration. Health systems implementing technologies to support pharmacy core processes including dispensing, preparation, and distribution took advantage of integration opportunities 60% of the time compared to 40% for technologies used to support ordering and administration.

Thirteen of 51 organizations polled indicated that they had implemented CPOE systems to support the ordering phase of medication management. However, only 7 of the 13 identified some level of integration with PIMS, with four reporting interoperability.

Thirty-five percent of respondents indicated implementing systems to support medication administration including smart pumps, BCMA, and electronic medication administration records. Sixty-five percent of the organizations polled had deployed smart pumps, representing a nearly 20% increase from a similar survey conducted in 2006; however, integration or interoperability with either pharmacy information or CPOE systems was absent in all cases. Any opportunity for automation and device integration or interoperability including dispensing cabinets, smart pumps, inventory management systems, and sterile IV compounding equipment was limited to pharmacy information management systems only. No information exchange or integration was reported between computerized physician order entry and electronic medical record (EMR) systems and distribution, preparation, or administration devices. Nearly 70% of respondents indicated that they had fully or partially implemented an EMR and roughly half of those indicated EMR or CPOE and decision support systems integration. Twenty percent of those polled indicated that they were currently working on deploying an EMR within the next year.

Fourteen percent of health systems indicated implementing systems to support all core medication management supporting processes (ordering, preparation, distribution, and administration) with only 6% indicating end-to-end integration. And, finally, 75% of organizations polled indicated implementing systems to capture pharmacy interventions with nearly all of them integrated with the pharmacy information system.

Conclusion

Current medication management supporting system deployment strategies have targeted and attempted to solve inefficiencies and error-prone practices within the boundaries of specific medication-use processes including ordering, transcribing, preparation, distribution, and administration. These single-threaded healthcare IT solutions have proven somewhat successful; however, many health systems have yet to realize the full potential of ideal medication management through the establishment of electronic data interchange and machine-interpretable data or interoperability. The benefits of physician ordering and pharmacy system integration have clearly been discussed in the literature including:

- The elimination of labor-intensive tasks
- Real-time medication order validation
- Reduction in medication-use cycle times
- Reduction in transcription errors[4]

Research surrounding medication errors and infusion pump technology indicated how these devices are integral for a safe medication management system, yet fall short in generating meaningful improvements in patient safety until they are interfaced with other systems, such as the EMR and CPOE systems.[5] To fully address the majority of medication-use system failures and sources for error, applications must be able to communicate and exchange data accurately, effectively, consistently, and multi-directionally with other medication and patient care–related systems, and, more importantly, they must be able to use the information exchanged. Medication-use system and automation integration allows for more effective and efficient communication of information across the medication-use process. By coupling integration with interoperability, health systems and providers are able to work together within and across organizational boundaries to advance the effective delivery of healthcare for individuals and communities.

Although this survey did not necessarily adhere to rigorous research principles, it did serve as a benchmark for those struggling to not only install medication management supporting systems but to also do it in an integrated way. This survey indicates that those health systems responding have yet to take advantage of medication-use process system integration or interoperability potentially leading to inefficient communication across the medication-use continuum and the introduction of new types of medication errors. The survey results clearly indicate that many health systems are effectively plugged in but have experienced limited success with connecting either through integration or interoperability. Despite significant advances and improvements with the deployment and use of these systems, it is clear that a great deal more work is necessary before ideal end-to-end medication management system integration and interoperability is achieved and the full potential realized.

References

1. Kohn LT, Corrigan JM, Donaldson MS, eds. To err is human: building a safer health system. Available at: www.nap.edu/catalog/9728.html. Accessed March 14, 2006.

2. Institute of Medicine Committee on Quality of Health Care in America. *Crossing the quality chasm: a new health system for the 21st century.* Washington, DC: National Academy Press; 2001.

3. Pedersen CA, Schneider PJ, Scheckelhoff DJ. ASHP national survey of pharmacy practice in hospital settings: prescribing and transcribing—2007. *Am J Health-Syst Pharm* 2008;65:827-843.

4. Bates DW, Cullen DJ, Laird N, et al. Incidence of adverse drug events and potential adverse drug events. Implications for prevention. ADE Prevention Study Group. *JAMA* 1995;274(1):29-34.

5. Husch M, Sullivan C, Rooney D, et al. Insights from the sharp end of intravenous technology medication errors: implications for infusion pump technology. *Qual Saf Health Care* 2005;14:80-86.

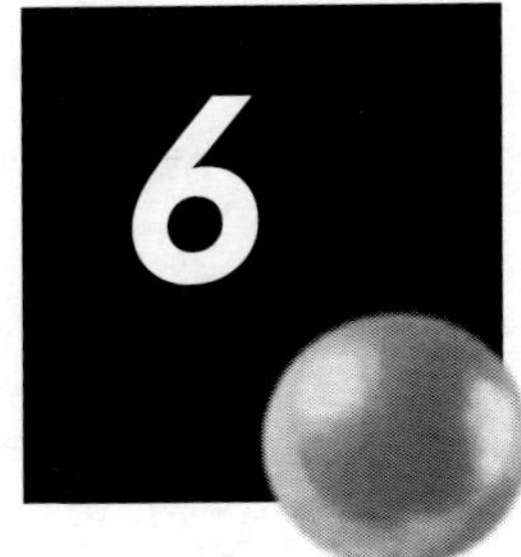

Downtime Bytes!

Patrice S. Johnson

Anywhere there are computers, there are downtimes. The Children's National Medical Center (CNMC) defines *downtime* as an interruption of the production system due to maintenance or upgrade (scheduled downtime) or unexpected system malfunction (unscheduled downtime).

Background

About 3 years ago, CNMC went live with an integrated system including computerized provider order entry, electronic medication administration record (eMAR), and Pharmnet. Since that time, we have also implemented modules to support nursing and physician documentation and medical records. As a result, we depend on our clinical system to be operational almost all of the time. It is essential for our clinicians to provide world-class service and care to our patients and their families. Therefore, the possibility of system downtime was something we were forced to consider at the planning stage of implementing such a robust clinical system.

Because safety is critical for us, we first implemented processes within the system to eliminate the occurrences of downtime. The goal was to have a reliable system with a 99% "uptime" in our production environment. High availability servers are what we have installed to help achieve this lofty goal. We still realize that scheduled and unscheduled downtimes are almost inevitable occurrences when computer-based operational systems are in place. However, CNMC has taken careful steps to outline a clear process and plan during downtimes that allows our staff to maintain an uninterrupted workflow without any compromise to the standard of care that is being delivered to our patients.

Goal of Downtime Process

- Maintain integrity of patient orders in the absence of clinical computer system
- Define a standardized process for converting patient orders to a paper ordering process
- Ensure timely patient orders and delivery of medications
- Define a process for managing the restart of the clinical computer system related to order entry
- Maintain integrity of medication administration documentation

Table 6.1. Methods Used for Staff Notification		
Notified via:	**Scheduled downtime**	**Unscheduled downtime**
Housewide e-mail	+	+
Clinical pager group	+	+
Inservices	+	
Computer splash screen	+	
Housewide signs	+	
Analyst unit notification		+

Downtime Notification Process

Communication is a key component to ensure a successful downtime process. All appropriate departments and individuals must be notified in a timely manner, whether the downtime is scheduled or unscheduled. However, when experiencing an unscheduled downtime, we have to rely on a fast, reliable means of getting the word out to our end-users as expeditiously as possible. One such method is having our analysts visiting or calling each unit and department to verbally notify the appropriate persons. Table 6.1 shows other methods utilized as means of staff notification.

Downtime Prep

After appropriate communication has been sent out, downtime preparation steps can begin. Many of the preparation steps involve the physician and the nurse as well as the pharmacist. In the event of a scheduled downtime, clinicians are asked to enter as many as orders as appropriate prior to the system going down. Nurses are asked to assess any missing doses that may be needed. The pharmacy is busy adhering to the above requests as well as a few other tasks listed below. A shared directory is used to house all necessary information related to downtime. This information is accessible by all pharmacy staff. A downtime kit is housed in the pharmacy which includes preprinted and blank labels for any orders that may come in during the downtime. The kit also includes additional information in case of an "extended" downtime or in the case of complete system failure. Such information includes blank eMars and labels for the typewriter. Of course, the preparation steps are omitted in the event of an unscheduled downtime.

Pharmacy Prep Steps

- Process incoming requests for medications
- Print eMars for nursing use
- Print patient profiles for pharmacy use
- Place Pyxis on override status
- Manually push out fill batches
- Disable all auto-print jobs
- Manually print all auto jobs (i.e., Therapeutic Drug Monitoring Report)

The System Is Down

During downtime, new orders and missing dose requests are submitted via fax. Our pharmacists use labels in a Word format to print the order. Many of our fast movers and standard concentrations are preprinted labels to help facilitate workflow. Staff has been educated to only request emergency medications during this period. Of course it's much easier to implement this plan during a scheduled downtime because clinicians can be reminded to write orders prior to the downtime. Pharmacists are required to document all orders for reconciliation purposes once the system is available. Much of the process while the system is down is typically uneventful if careful pre-downtime and post-downtime planning has been executed.

Downtime Support

Second to communication in being a key component to downtime success is adequate support. During scheduled downtime, we usually staff an extra pharmacist and two extra technicians pre-downtime and post-downtime to facilitate handling the peak in orders, phone calls, and requests that come in prior to the system being offline and right after the system is back up. The technician's role is vital for triaging phone calls and missing doses, while allowing pharmacist the time to focus on new medication orders. Technicians are also vital in sorting and delivering the eMars to each unit. Support from leadership, pharmacy management, and information technology management is also available when needed. Having adequate support is certainly of great comfort to those who happen to be on the frontline during downtime.

We Are Live!

Once the system becomes available, pharmacy is notified before that information is released to the house. It is our policy to enter all faxed orders into the system after we are back online. Pharmacy is given a period to "catch up." After pharmacists have entered all appropriate orders, nurses are then notified to reconcile the eMar with the printed medication administration records that were sent by pharmacy. If there are any discrepancies, pharmacy is notified. Once the reconciliation process is completed, the system is released housewide to our end-users.

Additional Resources

www.childrensnational.org
http://www.hmstn.com/technologies

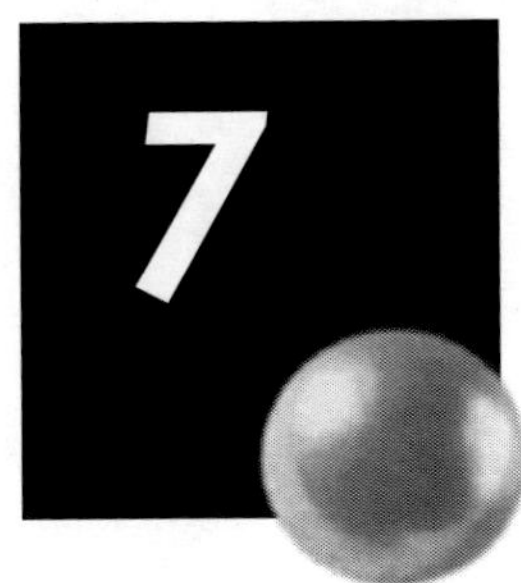

What Did You Do With My Medication?

Barbara L. Giacomelli

Background and Introduction

This chapter describes the process used to track a patient's personal supply of medication brought into the hospital from home. A patient's personal supply of medication is either stored in the pharmacy during the patient's encounter or identified and dispensed to the patient care area. The hospital, in accordance with regulatory standards, has a policy and procedure that allows patients to use their own supplies of medication during patient encounters, based on a prescriber's order if the medication is not on the hospital formulary.[1] The hospital had difficulty keeping track of patients' personal supplies of medication and developed a database within the pharmacy to ensure accurate tracking. The database has also provided valuable information on the types of medications a patient brings into the hospital and has also reduced hospital expenses related to reimbursing a patient for "lost" or "misplaced" personal medications.

Institution

Shore Memorial Hospital (SMH) is a nonprofit, community hospital located in southern New Jersey within a resort community. Opened in 1940, the hospital is licensed for 302 beds, operating with an average daily census of 180 patients. Services include adult medical and surgical, obstetrics, neonatal, and pediatrics. A priority patient care focus is neurology, oncology, orthopedics, nephrology, and cardiology. SMH operates two outpatient dialysis centers and several ambulatory clinics. SMH is an affiliate of the University of Pennsylvania Health System and the Children's Hospital of Philadelphia. A member of the national healthcare alliance, VHA, Inc., SMH contracts for supplies and pharmaceuticals through Novation. SMH is also an active member of the New Jersey Hospital Association. Patient safety through automation within the pharmacy and implementation of barcode medication administration (BCMA) have been part of process improvement initiatives engaged in over the past 3 years to improve inventory management and patient safety. Pharmacy services are highly automated with a robot for first dose and 24-hour cassette fill, automated dispensing cabinets for floor stock, and controlled substances and BCMA at the bedside. Pharmacists are decentralized for order entry and patient care rounds throughout the hospital for a minimum of 8 hours a day.

Concerns Regarding Patients' Personal Supplies of Medication

Prior to 2007, the pharmacy maintained a log form, manually tracking patients' personal medications sent to the pharmacy for storage or administration during patient encounters. These personal supplies were sent to the pharmacy through various mechanisms. They were either placed in the "Pharmacy Return Bin," located in each patient care area medication room, sent through the hospital pneumatic tube system, brought to the pharmacy window, or given to a pharmacy technician during routine medication delivery rounds. They arrived in brown paper bags, zip lock bags, laboratory specimen bags, and loose bottles. There were common instances in which the manual log did not match information the patient provided to his or her nurse, and the hospital was forced to reimburse patients for "lost medications." In addition to patient complaints, the pharmacy commonly found patients' personal medications being administered, during hospital encounters that had not been identified by the pharmacy, a regulatory violation.[2]

Goals for Tracking Patients' Personal Supplies of Medications

The goals for tracking patients' personal supplies of medication involved:

- Developing a computer database to track the patient's personal supply of medications electronically.
- Treating the patient's personal supply of medications as personal property, securing it at the bedside, so there wasn't a question regarding what medications were being sent to the pharmacy.
- Accurately tracking in the pharmacy when the patient's personal supply of medication was received and noting whether it was stored in the pharmacy or dispensed to the patient care area.
- Ensuring the pharmacy properly identified the patient's personal supply of medication before it was administered to the patient or notifying the patient's physician if unable to do so.
- Implementing a secure process for returning the patient's personal supply of medications at discharge.

Database Development

During a pharmacy staff meeting, the issues surrounding management of patients' personal supplies of medications were discussed. A pharmacy technician, proficient in Microsoft Access™, offered to develop a database for tracking patients' personal medications, incorporating these suggestions. The database, named "Personal Med Tracker" (Fig. 7.1) includes:

- Access for all pharmacy personnel and ease of use;

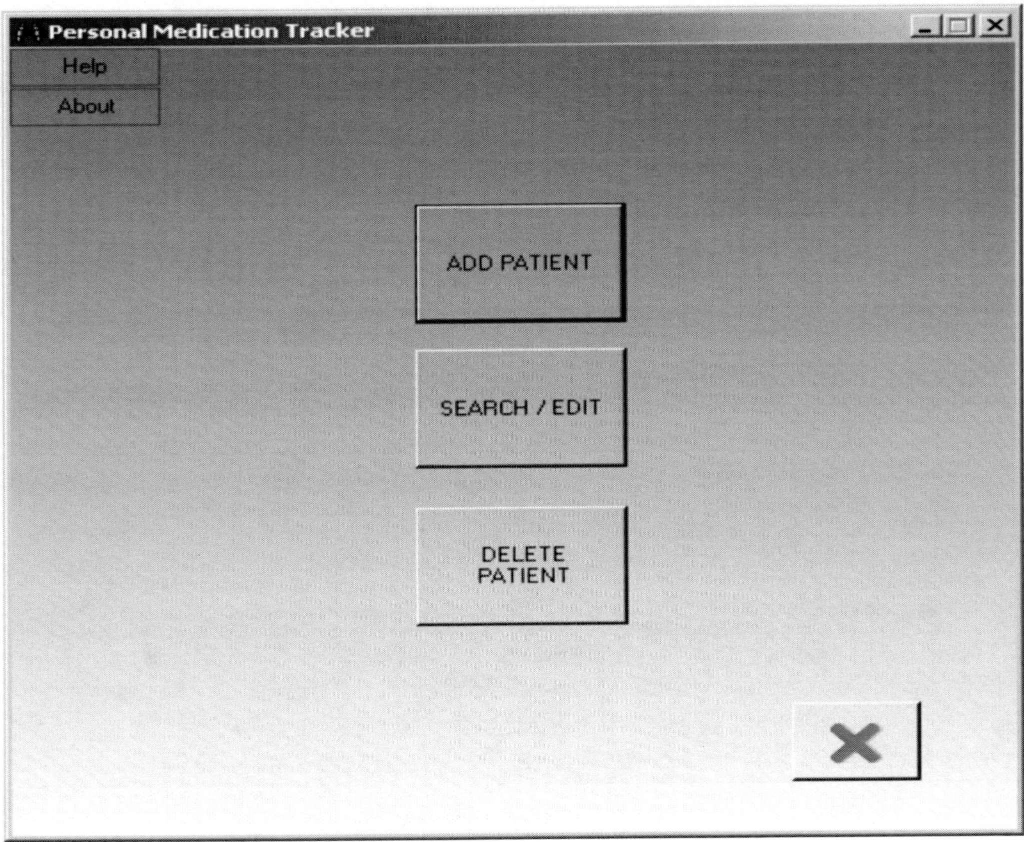

Figure 7.1. Personal Medication Tracker.

- Centralized location on one computer so data is only entered in one location;
- Tracked, searchable basic patient demographic information;
- Ability to enter data and edit data already entered;
- Medication tracking to show whether personal supply of medications are being stored in the pharmacy, dispensed to a patient care area, or sent back to the patient at discharge;
- Capability to generate reports to track and trend the data as needed or requested;
- Maintenance of historical information in the database for a minimum of 1 year.

Security and Storage of Patients' Personal Medications

To ensure security of a patient's personal supply of medications, the pharmacy worked with nursing to update the existing policy and procedure. Rather than allowing patients' personal supplies of medications to arrive in the pharmacy through different venues, the following was implemented (Fig. 7.2):

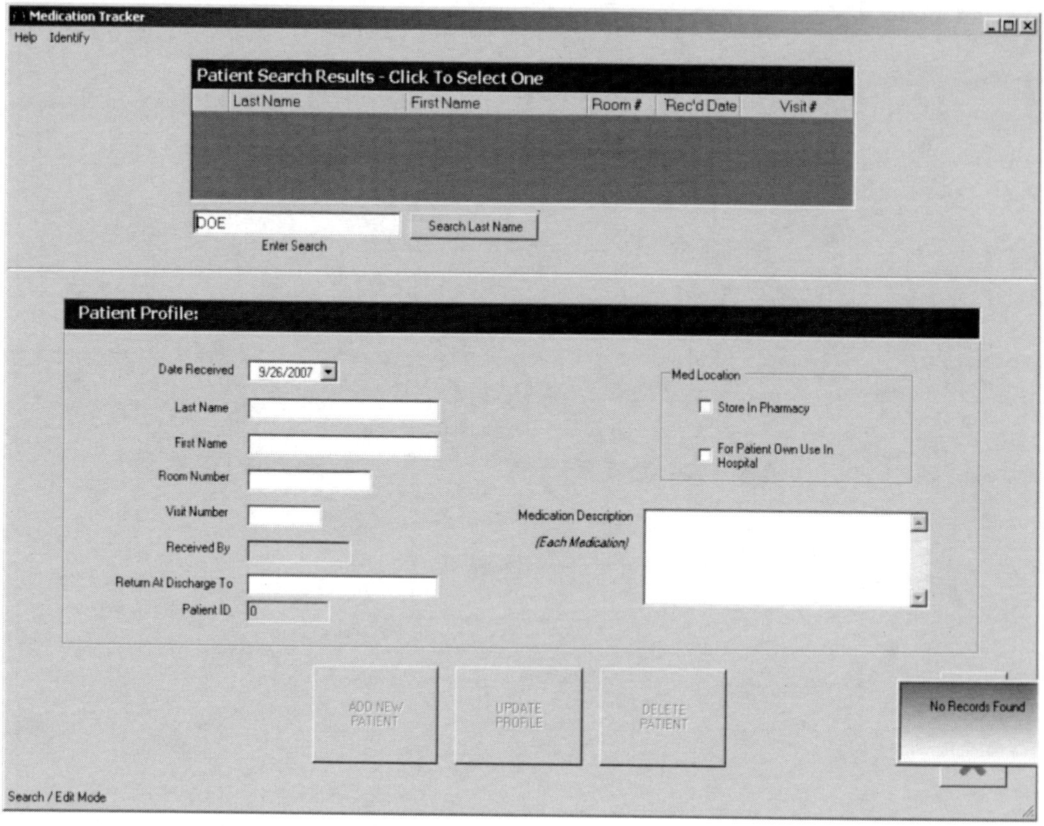

Figure 7.2. Patient profile medication tracker.

- A tamper-evident "medication security envelope" was purchased from a national supply vendor, which contains a numbered tear-away receipt.

- Nursing completes the required information on the envelope and secures the medications in the envelope in front of the patient and/or family members. This information includes:

  o Patient name

  o Encounter number

  o Room location

  o Medications removed from patient

- The numbered tear-away receipt is placed in the patient's chart, and the number corresponds to the envelope number sent to the pharmacy.

- The envelope is stored in the patient care area medication room (Pharmacy Return Bin) and is picked up by the pharmacy during routine medication rounds.

- Pharmacy logs the information in the database and stores the medication alphabetically in a designated area.

- Once the pharmacy receives a medication order indicating the patient "may use own supply," the pharmacist identifies the medication, applies an identification sticker, updates the database as well as the patient's medication profile, and dispenses to the patient care area.
- Upon discharge, the pharmacy is notified and returns any remaining medication from the patient's personal supply not used during the patient encounter directly to the nurse caring for the patient in the original security envelope. The pharmacy updates the database, noting that the medications have been returned.

Post-Implementation Follow-up

The database and medication security envelopes were implemented in January 2007. Since that time, the pharmacy has not had to replace any medications from a patient's personal supply. When inquiries occur, the pharmacy can easily view the database and locate the information. Patients are more comfortable releasing their personal supply of medications knowing they have been secured in tamper-evident envelopes in their presence. Limiting the drop-off location for a patient's personal supply of medications to the secured medication room in the patient care area has also minimized the opportunity for loss. Initially, there were requests to have the database available on multiple computers throughout the hospital but having the medications stored only in the pharmacy centralizes where inquiries are made.

There have been challenges such as when a patient's personal supply of a controlled substance is received because the procedure requires counting the contents of the patient's personal supply in front of the patient. These medications are then secured in the pharmacy controlled substance cabinet, which requires more steps for nursing and the pharmacy but is important from a security perspective. The pharmacy has requested that the database be updated to include the name of the pharmacy personnel documenting in the database so when questions arise the person accountable for logging the information and securing the medications can be easily identified.

Conclusion

The implementation of a database to track a patient's personal supply of medications and the updated policy and procedure have been well received by pharmacy, nursing, the medical staff, and patients. There is confidence in the process, and patient complaints are minimal. The database has also been used to track and trend the types of medications being authorized by prescribers as "patient take own." This data has been reported biannually to the Pharmacy and Therapeutics Committee, and the data have been used by the committee to complete several formulary class reviews. These formulary class reviews have resulted in formulary additions, formulary deletions, and therapeutic substitutions. The hospital has also begun distributing "Medication Pocket Cards" throughout the community to encourage patients to record their "home medication list" rather than bringing in their personal supply of medications when they come to the hospital.

References

1. Bing, CM. Compliance with the Joint Commission Medication Management Standards. In: *A Guide to JCAHO's Medication Management Standards.* Oakbrook Terrace, IL: Joint Commission Resources; 2006.
2. N.J.A.C. Title 8, Chapter 43G, Hospital Licensing Standards; 2005 with adoptions. http://www.state.nj.us/health/healthfacilities/documents/ac/njac43g_hoslicstd.pdf.

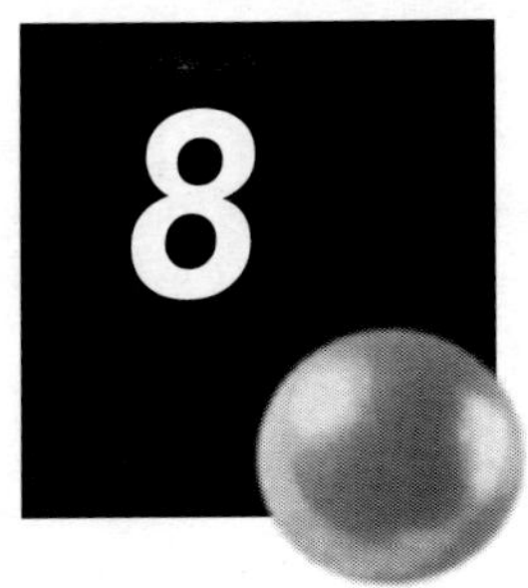

Barcodes: They're Not Just for Medication Administration Anymore

Lynn Ethridge

Background and Introduction

Greenville Hospital System University Medical Center (GHSUMC) is a nonprofit teaching and research institution nationally known for its advanced technology, comprehensive services, and outstanding staff. One of the largest health systems in the southeast and the only academic medical center in upstate South Carolina, GHSUMC comprises five medical campuses. The system has 1,146 beds, more than 1,000 affiliated medical staff, and 7,700 employees. Its seven residency programs provide training for 150 physicians. Additionally, three pharmacy residents along with more than 1,400 nursing and 300 allied health students receive clinical education within the system each year.

Greenville Memorial Hospital (GMH) is the state's largest acute care hospital with 750 beds. It contains Greenville's only 24-hour Level 1 trauma center and dedicated chest pain center, children's hospital and emergency department, pediatric intensive care unit (ICU), and highest level neonatal ICU. Its cardiac and women's services are the largest in South Carolina. Cancer, rehabilitation, behavioral health, and wellness services—all located on Greenville Memorial Medical Campus (GMMC)—are highly respected as well.

This chapter will review GMMCs process for ensuring safety by using barcode technology to dispense medications from the pharmacy department. One of the goals of the pharmacy department was to reduce the number of wrong medications dispensed to nursing; thus reducing the number of medication errors at the bedside.

In 2004, one of the organizational objectives of GHSUMC was to implement barcode medication administration (BCMA). The need to have medications with machine-readable barcodes was a necessity to make this project meaningful and successful. There was no Food and Drug Administration (FDA) mandate for manufacturers to provide unit-dose barcode medications. A review of the pharmacy inventory revealed that many medications had no barcode. The goal of the pharmacy department was to find a fast, efficient way to provide barcodes to unit dose medications.

Another goal of the pharmacy was to manage and automate the workflow of an extremely busy and complex centralized pharmacy distribution department. GMH pharmacy takes care of all hospitals located on the GMMC campus and, thus, provides medications to each of these facilities.

The pharmacy department began looking at different systems on the market to make the process of applying barcodes efficient. After months of research, Automed's family of hardware and software choices were chosen to help with these initiatives.

Description of the Filling Process

Barcodes on medications are used in a number of different areas within the pharmacy department to ensure correct dispensing of medications. The GMMC campus is currently 50% cart filled and 50% unit-base cabinet.

Orders are placed in the pharmacy order entry system from satellite pharmacies scattered throughout GMMC. The patient account number and the list of medications interface to multiple pieces of software located in the centralized filling area within GMH and to unit-based cabinets located on each nurse station.

Dispensing First Doses

Automed Workpath® is used to automate and track the workflow of first doses processed within a cart-fill environment. Computer screens alert technicians to new orders to be filled along with icons denoting the storage area within pharmacy where the item can be retrieved (Fig. 8.1).

Automed's FastPak EXP® is one area where medications are housed. This machine stores the top 300 medications that are ordered in bulk. Each canister contains a barcode associ-

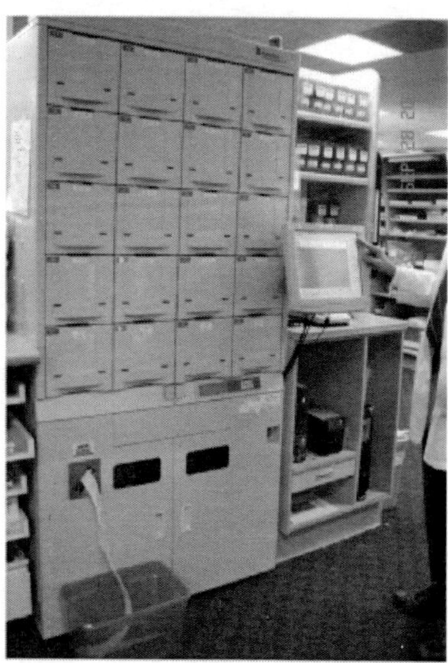
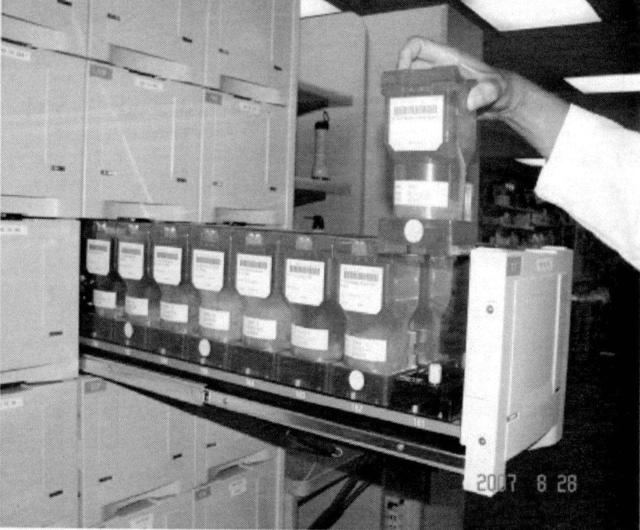

Figure 8.1. Automed Workpath.

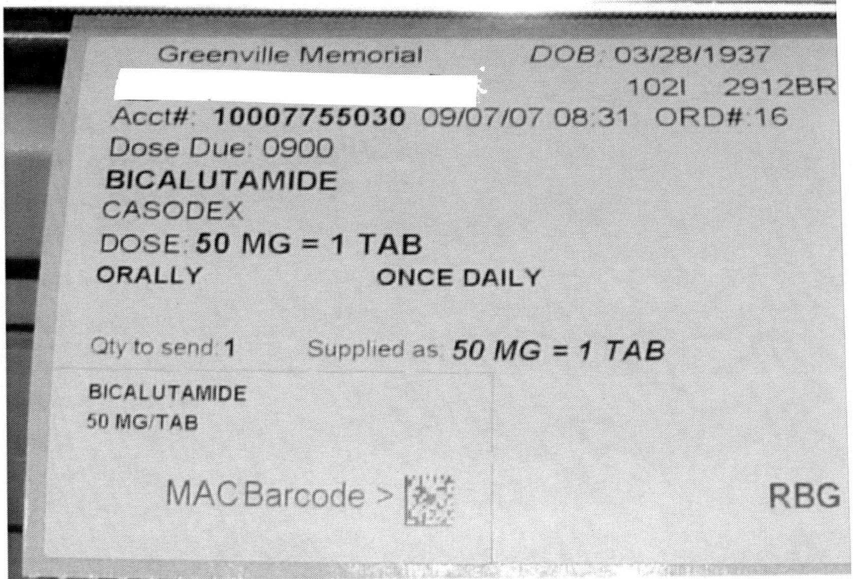

Figure 8.2. Sample of MAC barcode.

ated with a specific medication that the machine reads to correctly fill th
dose. The device produces a strip of unit dose medications in pouch packag
a barcode specific for each medication. The first package in the strip incl
name, room number, and account number with a barcode containing the p
number (Fig. 8.2). Next are the individual medications, and finally is a p
"last medication" for that patient.

Another area where medications are stored is in the carousels. GMH uses
Find® carousels. The technician picks the medication listed on the computer scre
rotates and lights up the area where the medication is stored. The medication
the barcode is scanned. A correct scan produces a patient-specific label that
medication for dispensing. An incorrect scan alerts the technician that the wr
was scanned and, thus, no label is produced.

Other areas of the pharmacy include the shelf or the refrigerator as deno
These areas are where unit-dose medications and bulk items too large for the car
Included are items that are unit-dose packaged and barcoded with a slower p
uses the Euclid Cadet and the Euclid Wet Cadet (Fig. 8.3).

The technician marks the computer screen to alert all others that the med
retrieval process (to avoid duplicate work). The medication is then scanned a
base. A correct scan produces a patient-specific label to place on the medicatio
scan alerts the technician that the wrong medication is being scanned; theref
not print. The labels are designed with a drug-specific barcode that is removal
the product has a manufacturer barcode. These software-produced barcodes a
liquids and topicals (useful for when tubes are crinkled after use). Lastly, the tech
the medication for a pharmacist's final check before sending to a nurse.

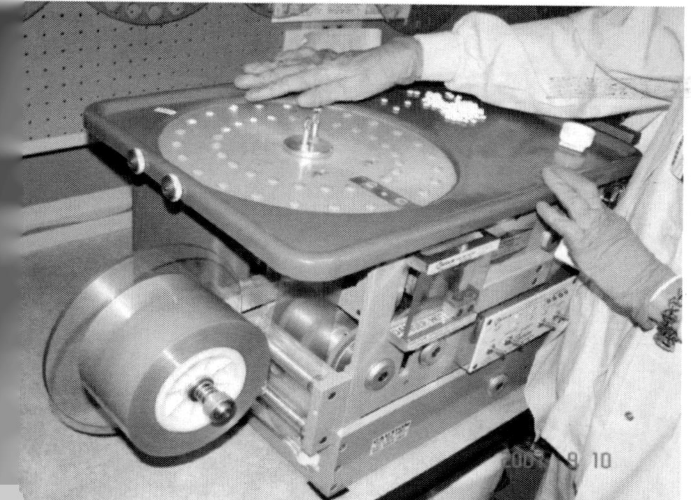
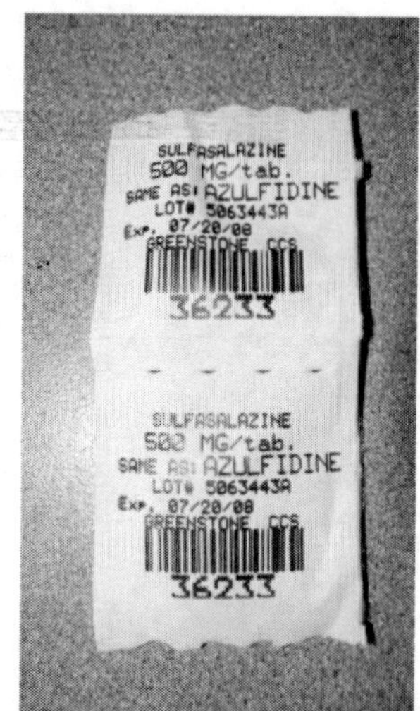
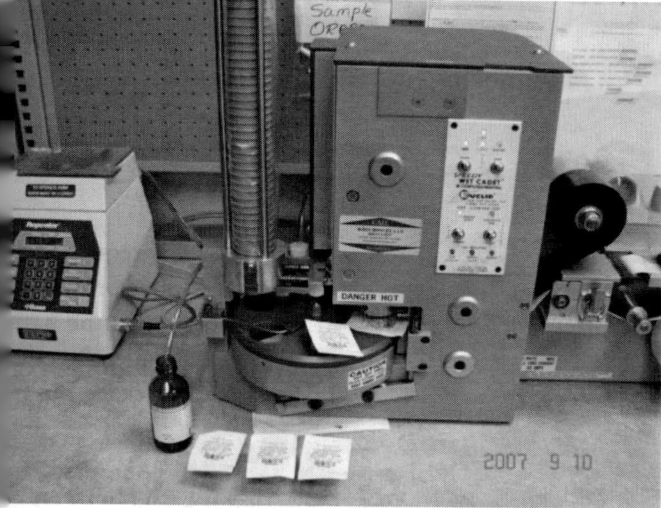
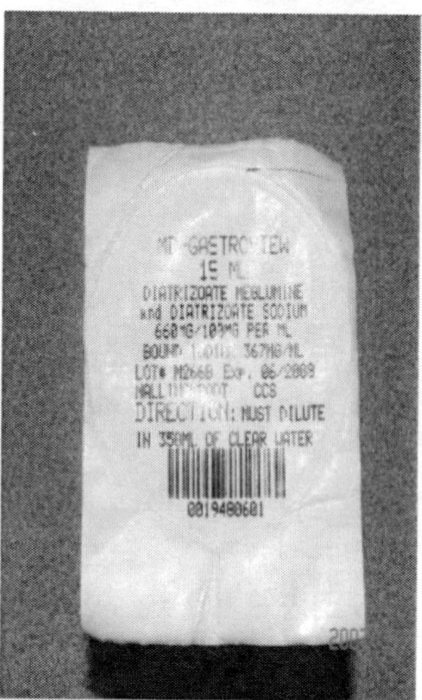

ure 8.3. Euclid Cadet and Euclid Wet Cadet systems and system-produced barcodes.

Pharmacist's Final Check

pharmacist performs a final check on each dose before sending it to the floor. Each label tains two barcodes. The pharmacy-use-only barcodes contain the patient's account number g with the corresponding medication order number. This barcode is scanned into the soft-e, whereby the patient and the list of medications to be dispensed are retrieved. The product code is then scanned against the appropriate medication to ensure proper dispensing. The ware additionally provides a picture of the medication as a second check to ensure that the per medication was indeed chosen to fill the order (Fig. 8.4).

The second barcode on the label, denoted as *MAC Barcode,* is specific to the medication. ontains either the national drug code number or the drug code listed in the pharmacy drug

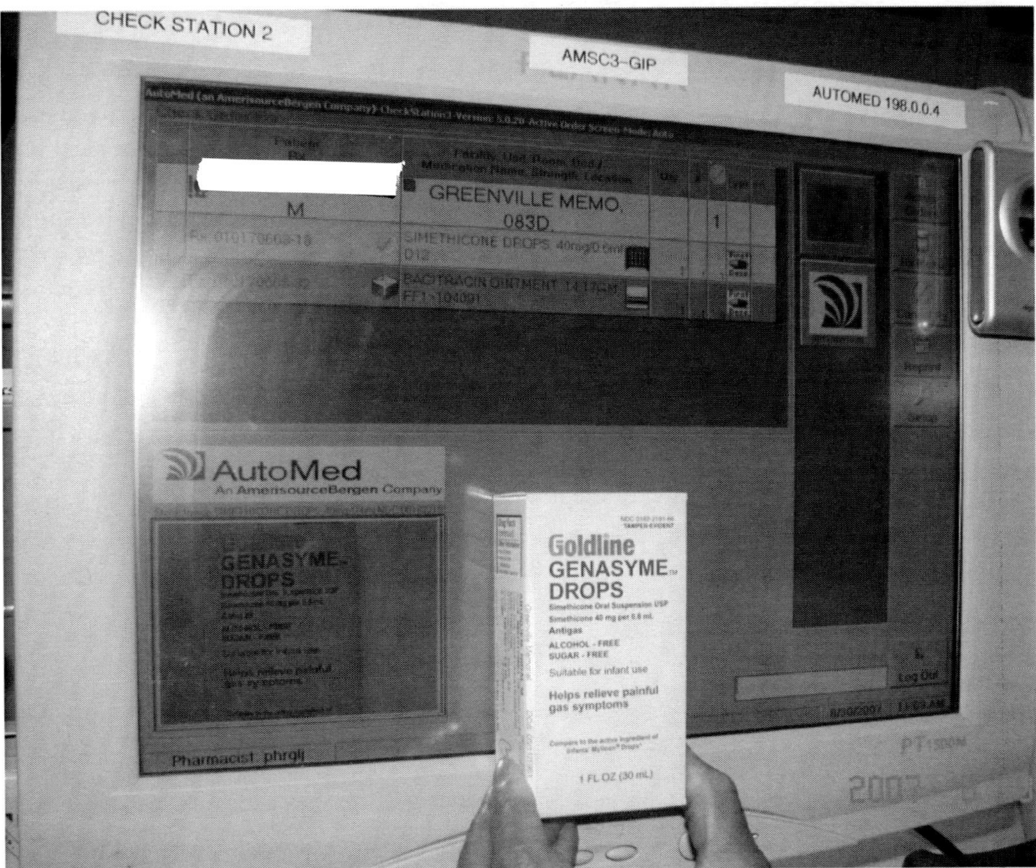

Figure 8.4. Barcode system check of proper medication.

master. This section of the label is perforated and removed before dispensing if the product contains a manufacturer barcode. Nurses use the MAC Barcode for scanning medications in the BCMA system for products that do not contain a manufacturer barcode.

Dispensing 24-hour Refills

About 50% of the GMMC campus is cart filled. A robot is used for this process and reads barcodes to pick the correct medication. A needs list is generated for a specific nurse station. Manufacturer-barcoded or internally barcoded unit-dose medications from the needs list are then loaded into the machine, whereby multiple scanners placed at various positions read the barcode from a conveyor belt. A robot arm then picks up the medication after it has been read and houses it in a compartment. The machine remembers the compartment location of each medication and retrieves it later for future dispensing into the medication cart.

Refilling Unit-based Cabinets

GHSUMC use barcode technology to fill and refill stock in the unit-based cabinets. Refill lists print with barcodes specific to each machine. Technicians scan the barcode on the refill list into the designated machine. The machine responds by lighting and opening each drawer and pocket associated with each medication printed on the refill list. We have found this feature to be a huge time saver for our technicians. The technician scans the medication and then the pocket to ensure that the correct medication is being placed in the proper location. This same functionality applies to nurses returning medications to a cabinet.

Conclusion

Barcode technology is used in many different ways within the pharmacy department to ensure proper dispensing of medications.

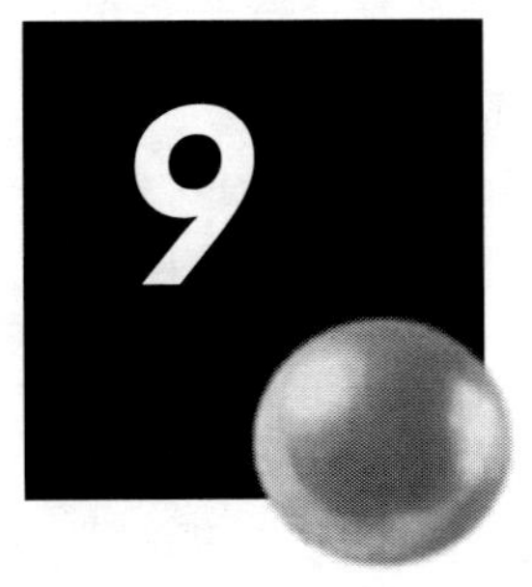

Using Genealogy Data Linked to Hospital Records to Build a Unique Pharmacogenomic Research Resource

Frederick S. Albright

Background and Introduction

Many genomic and genetic resources already exist to research genetic, familial, and environmental sources of disease throughout world and have been used with much scientific success. Some of these resources may also be valuable for the study of health-related or treatment-related phenotypes in pharmacogenomics, pharmacogenetics, metabolomics, and the other "omics." Knowledge about the heritability of medication response, as an example, could provide the beginnings of new and promising pharmacotherapeutic methods to better treat especially serious diseases of many types. Here we describe a larger generative data resource comprising other data resources, which could be analyzed with genetic epidemiological software tools to further our understanding of the genetic basis of host responses to medications.

A core unique resource created in Utah in the 1970s originally conceived by Mark Skolnick and colleagues,[1,2] continues to grow and provide the basic data for many studies of heritable predispositions to many disease phenotypes. This resource, the Utah Population Database (UPDB) was originally composed of genealogical records for the Utah population, linked to various electronic medical registries representing Utah. A unique set of customized software tools were created to examine evidence for excess familial cancer clustering among affected individuals by the Genetic Epidemiology Division in the Department of Biomedical Informatics, School of Medicine, at the University of Utah. This group continues to this day, and here I describe the present state of this resource and the unique analytical tools which are applied to the data for numerous genetic studies of human inheritance of diseases, with specific attention to the potential to apply these same methods to data for phenotypes related to medication response. I also describe important extant scientific research issues originating in collaboration, privacy and confidentiality, and policy unique to research projects of this type.

The Utah Genealogic Resource

The UPDB is a computerized genealogical research database originally created and maintained by Mark Skolnick, et al. in the 1970s.[1,2] The resource was originally designed to allow discovery of the genetic contribution to cancer.[3,4] The first set of diagnosis data linked to the Utah Genealogy was the Utah Cancer Registry, which has been a National Cancer Institute Surveillance, Epidemiology, and End-Result program registry since 1973. From its beginnings, the UPDB has been a valuable resource for numerous other projects.[5,6] The original genealogical records were obtained from the Utah Family History Library. The records came in the form of three-generation groupsheets that listed a couple, parents of each, and all offspring. These groupsheets were record-linked together as they were electronically entered. In 1982, this valuable biomedical science resource was ceded to the State of Utah and later to the University of Utah Resource for Genetic and Epidemiologic Research (RGE)[7-9] to manage and maintain. RGE adds new records yearly. These additions include new genealogic records added to the UPDB based on family triplet information from birth and death certificates (mother, father, and child) for Utah.

The UPDB includes a number of linked data resources, e.g., the Utah Cancer Registry, Utah driver license data, state-wide birth and death certificates, and, most recently, records of the electronic data warehouse (EDW) of the University of Utah Hospital and clinics, an electronic health record system.[9] Currently, the Genetic Epidemiology Division uses UPDB data for more than 2.2 million individuals, including Utah Mormon pioneers and their descendants, linked in genealogies that are 3 to 10 generations deep. The size and breadth of these genealogies provide greater power and utility in statistical discernment when linked to other data sources, e.g., as with the Utah Cancer Registry Records, in understanding genetic contributions to predispositions to cancer, given the greater detail of familial information.

Cancer

In addition to the discovery of evidence for genetic predisposition for a number of cancers,[10-12] the Genetic Epidemiology pedigree studies based on the UPDB cancer registry–linked data have had a critical and direct positive contribution in the discovery of cancer genes such as melanoma, prostate, and breast cancer.[13-15]

Other Diseases

Researchers have used the UPDB to discover and describe evidence for heritable predisposition to many different phenotypes. Recently the UPDB and death records have been used to report a heritable predisposition to death from viral influenza.[16] In this particular study, the software analysis tools developed by the Genetic Epidemiology Division were employed to discover and describe an infectious disease. Recently, a heritable predisposition has also been suggested for chronic fatigue syndrome using the UPDB linked to the electronic medical data warehouse using the same methodology.[17,18] Other published familiality studies using the UPDB and suggesting genetic predisposition include asthma mortality,[19] diabetes,[20] aneurysm,[21] and chronic kidney failure.[22] Many other research projects use the UPDB resource; their publications are available on the UPDB website.

So, as biomedical research scientists we ask, "can the UPDB resource be repurposed, extended, and refined to discover and understand significant host medication responses ultimately originating from host genetics? Further, can we also begin to more fully understand the interaction of host genetics and epigenetics through using the UPDB? Let's examine the proposed methodology.

Methodology

Briefly, in the interest of economy, I would like to give the general overview of the methodology. As with the cancer studies, it begins with linking records of the necessary type with the UPDB.

Electronic Data Warehouse Records Linked to the Utah Population Database

Individuals within the UPDB have been linked to patient information from the University of Utah Hospitals and Clinics EDW.[9] A total of 1.5 million patients were successfully linked from the EDW to the UPDB. This linkage creates the infrastructure for research projects to access medical information if they have the appropriate Institutional Review Board (IRB) and RGE permissions. Records within the EDW include diagnosis and procedure coding as well as prescription and laboratory test results.

Defining the Familial and Genetic Component of Disease

Diseases can be modeled on a causal continuum from purely genetic to purely environmental (could be familial due to proximity or common exposure but not heritable genetics). Responses to medication are also most likely due to interactions between genes and environment. Studies of the heritable response to medications clearly require the environmental insult of exposure to a specific medication, combined with a predisposition to a specific response to such exposure, and could be further confounded by the necessary co-aggregation of the condition requiring treatment with a specific medication.

There are three methods that we typically apply to explore the familial nature of phenotypes. These three methods of analysis are (1) estimation of relative risks in relatives, (2) a test for excess relatedness, and (3) identification of high-risk pedigrees.

Estimation of Relative Risk in Relatives

If a specific medication response has a heritable component, then it follows that the same or similar medication response should occur at a higher frequency among similarly exposed relatives of the cases compared to random controls. For estimation of relative risk, we compare the rate of the medication response phenotype in exposed relatives of cases with the rate of the medication response in exposed individuals in the Utah population. We have historically used rates estimated internally from the UPDB; for studies described here, we use a different but similarly rigorous methodology, which will be discussed later in this monograph.

Analysis of Familiality

We use the Genealogical Index of Familiality (GIF) to test the hypothesis of no excess relatedness in individuals with the phenotype of interest.[23-24] The GIF analysis measures the average relatedness of all possible pairs of cases, using the Malécot coefficient of kinship.[25] The coefficient of kinship for two individuals is the probability that two randomly homologous genes selected from each individual are identical by descent from a common ancestor. The coefficient is calculated by considering all paths of common descent. The coefficient of kinship for a pair of siblings is 1/4th; for uncle and nephew, 1/8th. The coefficient is smaller for more distant pairs of relatives. The GIF statistic (case GIF), or average relatedness of the case pairs, is then calculated as the mean coefficient of all possible pairs within the set of cases, and is multiplied by 10^5 for ease of comparison.

The test of the hypothesis for excess familiality within a group of cases is assessed by comparing the case GIF to the control GIF distribution. For a single control GIF measurement, we select a set consisting of one control randomly selected from the UPDB to match each case by sex, birthplace (Utah or not), and 5-year birth cohort. The control GIF is determined in an analogous manner to the case GIF. The significance of the hypothesis test of no excess relatedness for cases is empirically based on the position of the case GIF in the distribution of the GIF values for the 1,000 matched control sets. This type of average-relatedness methodology originated with the Utah Genetic Epidemiology Division, but similar algorithms have been developed and employed by other groups, e.g., deCODE Genetics in Iceland.[26]

Conceptually, the GIF test measures the average relatedness of cases and compares it to the average relatedness expected in the population (based on multiple sets of matched controls). If a phenotype has a genetic component, then we would expect that the cases would be more closely related to each other than randomly selected controls. However, the GIF test cannot differentiate between excess familial clustering that is due to genes from excess familial clustering from shared environmental factors. We therefore also perform the GIF test while ignoring all close relationships observed. If the familial relationships observed between cases are only in excess for close relationships, then common environment cannot be ruled out.

If relationships for cases compared to controls are observed in excess for both close and distant relatives, a heritable genetic component to phenotype is strongly suggested.

Comparison of the contribution to the GIF statistic by the degree of relationship, for cases versus controls, allows identification of the relationships contributing most to the GIF statistic. For a disorder with no familial effect at all we would expect the case and control GIF distributions not to differ significantly. For a disease with a familial, but nongenetic effect, we would expect to see excess only among close relatives, because behavioral or environmental factors would primarily result in an excess of close relatives. For a disease with a genetic contribution, we would expect to see an excess of both close and distant relative pairs in cases versus controls.

High-risk Pedigrees

With the above tools, it is relatively easy to identify pedigrees in which an excess of members exhibit a medication-response phenotype. We hypothesize that such pedigrees are those most likely to represent a heritable predisposition to inappropriate medication response. In these pedigrees, positional cloning studies can be performed to map the medication response phenotype to a particular chromosomal locus. If a genetic region is identified, candidate genes in the region can be screened. Gene discovery follows if polymorphisms related to the host response phenotype segregating in the pedigree are identified.

Proposed Analysis of Response to Medication Phenotypes

Definition of Phenotypes

At this point, informatics analysis needs to be performed to define the medication response phenotypes to be studied. What defines a host medication-response phenotype to a particular medication? Given the number of medications and possible variability in responses, this will be a constant process, especially as the data representations evolve. Defining phenotypes associated with medication response is a significant scientific problem to be solved before familiality analysis can be done with certainty. In a sense, we are at a similar point in using the UPDB of almost 30 years ago when it was first applied to the discovery of heritable genetic contributions to the development of cancer.

Proposed Gene Identification and Gene Expression Studies Leading to Genetic Screening

High-risk pedigree studies are proposed to identify genes predisposing to an individual's medication response. Informative individuals in high-risk pedigrees are recruited, and blood is sampled for DNA (with patient official recorded consent and IRB and Health Insurance Portability and Accountability Act [HIPAA] approval). DNA samples are genotyped for markers representing the entire human genome. Linkage analysis of these markers in the high-risk pedigrees can identify markers that cosegregate with the phenotype of interest. From identification of the chromosomal locus of a hypothesized predisposition gene, molecular genetics studies can lead to gene identification and to discovery of the polymorphisms of the gene responsible for the medication-response phenotype observed. Molecular studies, such as metabolomics, are then done to further understand the role of the gene in response to the medication. From here the knowledge and information might be used to design and implement an FDA-approved genetic screening test in order to identify the risk of an inappropriate drug response of the medically implicated set of related medications. From the results, it should be possible in a number of cases to choose the best drug for the patient based on risk of a drug misadventure or reduced or increased medical efficacy balanced against the cost of the utilizing the medication in the individual. The goal is to increase the effectiveness of the medication prescribed and used, both in terms of health outcomes, to improve health at the lowest price to the individual. Ultimately, at the core of this process is medical efficacy and medication safety—increase the efficacy and lower the risk as appropriately measured against the other factors of the person and the disease.

Conclusion

The Genetic Epidemiology group has undertaken new research in a prototypic attempt to understand host medication-response contributions based on host genetics at the phenotypic level. So far, this looks as promising as our other UPDB research has been, as applied in previous studies enumerated in the bibliography at the end of this paper. However, there are meaningful scientific challenges as well that find their origins in collaboration, privacy, confidentiality, and policy, and there are technical and biomedical research issues involved in projects of this type. Let's examine some of these in the context of our current research and future research in pharmacogenomics.

Analysis Issues and Limitations

Automatic identification of the individuals who have a specific medication-response phenotype of interest from the electronic health record (EHR) is a critical issue for familiality analyses. Often one single piece of data, such as an International Classification of Diseases diagnosis code, cannot adequately identify the phenotype of interest in an individual. In future it may be possible to build methods to identify the phenotypes from the EHR, perhaps using computerized discrimination or decision logic, an example of the interface of science and technology.

The linked files of UPDB and the medical information from the University of Utah health system have a limitation based on censoring of all observations prior to 1994 in the EHR. Similarly, there is the censoring of phenotype data for patients treated outside the University of Utah system. Individuals whose genealogy is not represented in the UPDB or who do not record-link to their genealogy are also censored. Inaccuracies in genealogy data, resulting in incorrect assumptions being made about genetic relationships between cases, may also occur.

In general, it can be assumed that such censoring as occurs does so in an unbiased fashion and, therefore, perhaps only makes the tests of hypotheses performed more conservative in nature.

Because of the sensitive and private nature of the hospital phenotype data, it is not possible to have access to all hospital patient data at this time. This limitation makes selection of a larger set of appropriate matched controls difficult in terms of randomness, sample size, and matching.

Observations on the Social Interactions with the Scientific Studies

The interplay and dynamics of the legal, social, scientific, and technical issues can be engineered for scientific efficacy, with oversight agencies as HIPAA, IRB, and RGE. Patience, thought, and tolerance are required; the oversight agencies can play pivotal roles as "collaborative stewards" in providing appropriate access and services that enable scientific research and discovery in as unbiased a fashion as possible with reasonable levels of risk to the data resources under stewardship. These oversight individuals and groups play a comprehensively core role to manage the legal, policy, privacy, and cyber-threat risks to the patients and subjects, employees, and the parent institution for resources of the type discussed here, even if the records are anonymous or de-identified. Fostering the collaborative and stewardship relationships between the researchers and these agencies by the parent institution(s) would have a positive and beneficial effect on general research efficiency and perhaps be essential to the reduction in the costs of performing research, stretching the dwindling research dollars.

As scientists, we make every attempt to design our experiments to eliminate bias; otherwise, unscientific results occur and we reach unwarranted conclusions. We, too, must be stewards of the data resources at our disposal and collaboration is essential. If the oversight agencies understand the facts, data requirements, hypotheses, methods, and significance of the research, their actions in regard to requests for access to resources germane to the research can be unbiased. With that context, committees of oversight actually can become stewards that work with the researchers to enable safe, secure, low-liability, and privacy-protecting scientific research. Researchers in kind can more fully respond to the additional responsibilities for scientific stewardship of the data that is unbiased. Unbiased health research is as important as protecting the privacy and consent of data contributors. Transparency should be a goal between researcher and oversight committees, if not a culture.

Acknowledgments

This work was supported in part by the National Library of Medicine R01 LM009331 to LACA. Partial support for all datasets within the Utah Population Database was provided by the University of Utah Huntsman Cancer Institute. The author would like to gratefully acknowledge collaboration with the University of Utah, School of Medicine, the Department of Biomedical Informatics, Genetic Epidemiology Division (including Jim Farnham Statistical Analyst, Craig Teerlink Ph.D. candidate, Steven Backus, applications programmer, database and systems administrator, and the scientific leadership by the Genetic Epidemiological Director, Lisa Cannon-Albright).

References

1. Skolnick M, Bean L, Dintelman S, et al. A computerized family history database system. *Sociol Social Res* 1979;63:506-523.

2. Skolnick M. The Utah genealogical database: a resource for genetic epidemiology. In: Cairns J, Lyon JL, Skolnick M, eds. Banbury Report No 4; *Cancer Incidence in Defined Populations.* New York: Cold Spring Harbor Laboratory; 1980:285-297.

3. Cannon-Albright LA. Utah family-based analysis: past, present, and future. *Hum Hered* 2008;65:209-220.

4. Cannon-Albright LA, Skolnick MH, Bishop DT, et al. Common inheritance of susceptibility to colonic adenomatous polyps and associated colorectal cancers. *N Engl J Med* 1988;319(9):533-7.

5. Skolnick M, Bean L, May D, et al. Mormon demographic history I. Nuptiality and fertility of once-married couples. *Popul Studies* 1978;32:5-19.

6. McLellan T, Jorde L, Skolnick M. Genetic distances between the Utah Mormons and related populations. *Am J Hum Genet* 1984;36:836-837.

7. Resource for Genetic and Epidemiological Research, University of Utah. Homepage and overview. Available at: http://www.research.utah.edu/rge/. Accessed April 24, 2008.

8. Wylie JE, Mineau GP. Biomedical databases: protecting privacy and promoting research. *Trends Biotechnol* 2003;21:113-116.

9. University of Utah Population and Pedigree Resource: Utah Population Database. Homepage. Available at: http://www.hci.utah.edu/groups/ppr/index.html. Accessed April 24, 2008.

10. Skolnick M, Bishop D, Carmelli D, et al. A population-based assessment of familial cancer risk in Utah Mormon genealogies. In Arrighi FE: *Genes, Chromosomes, and Neoplasia.* New York, NY: Raven Press; 1980.

11. Bishop DT, Skolnick M. Genetic epidemiology of cancer in Utah genealogies: a prelude to the molecular genetics of common cancers. In: *Cellular and Molecular Biology of Neoplasia,* eds. Mak, TW and Tannock, I. *J Cell Phys* 1984;3(Suppl):363-377.

12. Cannon-Albright LA, Thomas A, Goldgar DE, et al. Familiality of cancer in Utah. *Cancer Res* 1994;54:2378-2385.

13. Miki Y, Swensen J, Shattuck-Eidens D, et al. A strong candidate for the breast and ovarian cancer susceptibility gene BRCA1. *Science* 1994;266(5182):66-71.

14. Kamb A, Shattuck-Eidens D, Eeles R, et al. Analysis of the p16 (CDKN2) as a candidate for the chromosome 9p melanoma susceptibility loci. *Nat Genet* 1994;8:22-26.

15. Tavtigian SV, Simard J, Teng DH, et al. A candidate prostate cancer susceptibility gene at chromosome 17p. *Nat Genet* February 2001;27(2):172-180.

16. Albright FS, Orlando P, Pavia AT, et al. Evidence for a heritable predisposition to death due to influenza. *J Infect Dis.* Jan 2008;197(1):18-24.

17. Albright F, Cannon-Albright L. Genetic contribution to chronic fatigue syndrome (CFS) and associated pain- and fatigue- related diagnoses described in a population-based genealogical resource in Utah. Presentation at: 8th International IACFS Conference on Chronic Fatigue Syndrome, Fibromyalgia and other Related Illnesses; January, 2007; Ft. Lauderdale, Florida.

18. Cannon-Albright LA, Albright FS. Evidence for a heritable component to chronic fatigue syndrome. Presentation at: 25th Annual American Pain Society Meeting; May, 2006; San Antonio, TX.

19. Teerlink CC, Hegewald MJ, Cannon-Albright LA. A genealogical assessment of heritable predisposition to asthma mortality. *Am J Respir Crit Care Med* 2007;176:865-870.

20. Weires MB, Tausch B, Haug PJ, et al. Familiality of diabetes mellitus. *Exp Clin Endocrinol Diabetes* November 2007;115(10):634-640.

21. Cannon Albright LA, Camp NJ, Farnham JM, et al. A genealogical assessment of heritable predisposition to aneurysms. *J Neurosurg* 2003;99(4):637-643. Related Articles, OMIM (calculated), Cited in PMC, LinkOut.

22. Goldfarb-Rumyantzev AS, Cheung AK, Habib AN, et al. A population-based assessment of the familial component of chronic kidney disease mortality. *Am J Nephrol* 2006;26(2):142-148.

23. Hill JR. A kinship survey of cancer in the Utah Mormon population. Ph.D. Thesis, University of Utah, Salt Lake City, Utah. 1980.

24. Hill JR: A survey of cancer sites by kinship in the Utah Mormon population. In: Cairns J, Lyon JL, Skolnick M, eds. Banbury Report No 4; *Cancer Incidence in Defined Populations.* New York: Cold Spring Harbor Laboratory; 1980:299-318.

25. Malécot G. *Les Mathematiques de L'heredite.* Paris, France: Masson; 1948.

26. Sveinbjornsdottir S, Hicks AA, Jonsson T, et al. Familial aggregation of Parkinson's disease in Iceland. *New Engle J Med* 2000;343:1765-1770.

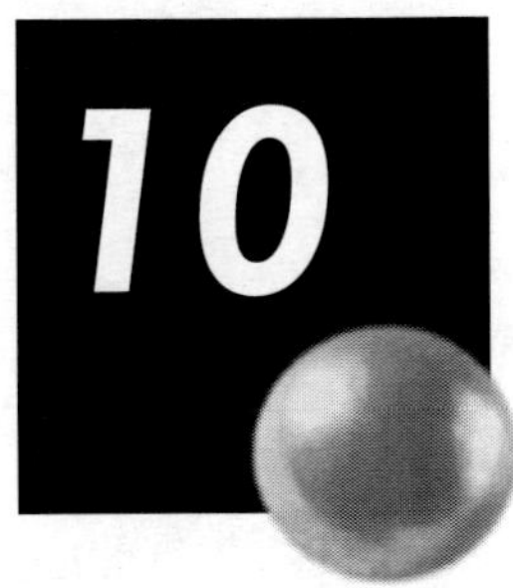

"If You Didn't Document It" . . . That's Old News

Brent I. Fox

Georgia W. Fox

Background and Introduction

Pharmacy has undergone a transformation: from a profession in the 1800s focused on medication compounding and the distribution of patent medications to today's focus on medication-related patient outcomes. *Clinical pharmacy* was the term introduced to describe a new approach to practice in the 1960s.[1,2] This process-oriented practice is focused on pharmacist-provided services intended to ensure safe and effective medication therapy. Services included pharmacokinetic dosing and antibiotic usage studies.[3] Additional clinical pharmacy activities included unit-dose distribution, medication-error monitoring and research, and involvement in pharmacy and therapeutics committees.[1,2,4] The net result of clinical pharmacy activities has been a change in pharmacists' focus from production of medications to activities that ensure safe and effective medication usage. Clinical pharmacy remains a strong component of pharmacy practice.

Today, pharmaceutical care is the mantra of pharmacy practice. Defined as, "the responsible provision of drug therapy for the purpose of achieving definite outcomes that improve a patient's quality of life," pharmaceutical care extends clinical pharmacy from a service-oriented practice to a patient-oriented practice in which the pharmacist shares responsibility for the patient's overall well-being.[5] The key distinction between clinical pharmacy and pharmaceutical care is the pharmacist's acknowledged covenant with the patient to ensure optimal medication-related outcomes.[6] "Care" is the core of pharmaceutical care; it signifies a greater commitment between the pharmacist and patient.

A primary component of pharmaceutical care is documentation of care provided.[6,7] The term "intervention" has been used to describe clinical pharmacy services, pharmaceutical care activities, and the actual documentation of these activities.[8,9] Although an authoritative definition for "intervention" in the context of pharmaceutical care has yet to be published, the term is widely recognized as pharmacists' documentation of care provided. In the decades since the 1960s, hundreds of published articles have described pharmacists' documentation of clinical interventions.[10] Table 10.1 contains a brief list of reasons for documenting interventions.

As clinical pharmacy and pharmaceutical care have become ingrained in the practice of pharmacy, the adage "if you didn't document it, you didn't do it," has become increasingly

Table 10.1. Reasons for Documenting Pharmaceutical Care Activities

1. Patients benefit when all caregivers are aware of pharmacists' activities.

2. Other patients benefit when pharmacists are able to draw upon knowledge learned through review of previous patient encounters.

3. Pharmacists benefit by being able to provide objective data about outcomes due to the care they provide.

4. Documentation provides a method for performance evaluation.

5. Documentation provides evidence of financial impact of pharmacy services.

6. Documentation provides an audit trail.

7. Healthcare payers benefit by pharmacists' activities that optimize medication use, ultimately decreasing overall healthcare costs.

important. Documented evidence of pharmacist-provided services and outcomes due to pharmacist-managed medication therapy is essential to demonstrate the pharmacist's role in patient care. Recognizing the importance of intervention documentation, institutional pharmacy leadership has consistently sought the best intervention documentation method.[11] Efforts have focused on selecting and implementing an electronic documentation method to replace manual, paper-based documentation systems.

Today, many pharmacy departments are beyond the "if you didn't document it" stage. Documentation systems have been implemented, and the focus is now on optimizing the documentation process. Auburn University Harrison School of Pharmacy (AUHSOP) is a publicly funded pharmacy program in Auburn, Alabama, offering PharmD, MS, and PhD degrees. Pharmacy practice faculty members are located throughout Alabama, and rotation sites are located in five southeastern states. After evaluating several intervention documentation systems, AUHSOP selected Quantifi® from Pharmacy OneSource for intervention documentation by pharmacy practice faculty members and students on rotations (clerkships). Through our evaluation, implementation, and use processes, we have identified many considerations for intervention documentation.

First Step: Build or Buy?

The obvious first step of selecting an intervention documentation system is one of the most important steps ultimately influencing your ability to optimize that system to your individual usage. Individual features and functions, and their impact on system administration and usage, are discussed. At this point, the initial choice of which system to implement ultimately influences the topics found. The first question you will be presented with is whether to buy a commercial documentation system or to use internal resources to develop your own documentation system.

Commercial systems are available from a variety of vendors, and these systems are specifically targeted for use in institutional settings (see Table 10.2). These systems are usually developed with pharmacist input and often fit reasonably well into pharmacy workflow. They are Internet-based and exist external to pharmacy management systems. Alternatively, many pharmacy management systems have intervention modules that can be an additional component to existing software. An obvious advantage of this approach is that the intervention module will interface with records within the pharmacy management system. A commercially available application that is not provided by your pharmacy management system vendor will also likely be able to exchange admission, discharge, and transfer data to provide a minimum dataset necessary for documentation.

The second method for acquiring documentation software is to build your own. Several options exist for this approach. The first option is to have the institution's information systems (IS) personnel build a custom documentation system that you design. They will likely be able to build a documentation tool that exchanges information with your pharmacy management system and is customized based on your specifications. A potential obstacle to this approach is the availability and willingness of IS personnel to meet your needs in a suitable timeframe. As you probably know, your relationship with IS can have a significant impact on this process.

The second approach to building an intervention documentation system is to build it yourself. Commercially available tools exist that allow users to build a database (see Table 10.3). Through the use of these tools, non-technically savvy individuals can build intervention documentation systems. The sophistication and capabilities of these self-built documentation tools are typically less than that found in commercially available applications. However, like the intervention documentation tool built by your IS staff, a tool you build will likely be customized to your individual needs.

Advantages and disadvantages exist for all potential options for developing an intervention documentation system. As with all decisions impacting the pharmacy department, careful

Table 10.2. Commercial Intervention Documentation Software

Name	Web site URL
Clini-Doc	www.clini-doc.com
PharmDoc.Net	www.mccreadiegroup.com
Quantifi	www.pharmacyonesource.com
RxRounds Interventions	www.medkeeper.com
TheraDoc Intervention Assistant	www.theradoc.com

Table 10.3. Database Development Software

Name	Web site URL
abcDB Database	www.pocketsoft.ca
HanDBase	www.ddhsoftware.com
PenDragon Forms	www.pendragon-software.com
SprintDB Pro	www.kaione.com
Visual CE	www.syware.com

consideration should be given to this decision. Regardless of the route chosen, an intervention documentation system will require some amount of financial resources. Even an application developed internally by IS personnel has the indirect cost of their development time and your time spent designing and working with IS.

Step Two: User Management

Prior to clinicians' use of the documentation tool, the system administrator is responsible for preparing the tool for use. One of the first preparation steps is the creation and definition of user role types. Role types determine permissions within the system, granting different roles access to different components and functions within the system. This is a key consideration for documentation systems. Institutions may have very different needs for roles, ranging from the total number of roles needed to the permissions that the "technician" role, for example, can perform. Will all users be able to access all other users' submitted data? Will all users be able to print all reports? Which user(s) will be able to manage user accounts? These and other questions must be answered. As you evaluate the options for a documentation tool, convene a planning group to thoroughly discuss your unique needs regarding roles and carefully examine the available systems to ensure their roles management capabilities meet your needs.

Once user roles are defined, depending on the size of the institution and user base, adding, modifying, or deleting user accounts can require a significant amount of time and resources. Batch processing of users—whether adding, modifying, or deleting accounts—provides an efficient method to handle user management. Account management at the individual user level remains a necessary function, but for larger institutions or situations in which users' accounts are acted on at the same time, batch processing is beneficial.

From the perspective of the system administrator, account functions, such as responses to username and password reminder requests, should be automated to the fullest extent possible. Users forget their login information, and they often need this information at the moment they begin to document an intervention. User requests for login information should be able to be processed without system administrator action. The system administrators will benefit because they can devote their time to more complex and higher impact system oversight activities. More importantly, users benefit for automated processing of these requests because they will not have to wait on administrators to handle the requests. It is likely that the documentation administrator will have other responsibilities and may, in fact, be one of the clinical pharmacy staff members. It is unlikely that the documentation administrator will be sitting in front of a computer the majority of the time waiting on users' requests for help.

Step Three: Speed, Speed, Speed

As with other clinical information systems like computerized prescriber order entry, one of the most important considerations for integrating documentation into a clinician's workflow is the impact the documentation system has on the clinician's time. A slow, labor-intensive documentation system is a tool that will ultimately not be used. Numerous methods are available to create efficient documentation systems, beginning with the user's initial login.

Although it seems obvious, careful consideration should be given to the amount of steps, or "clicks," required for a clinician to access a documentation system. Access time is minimized in systems that are integrated with a pharmacy management system in which the clinician is already logged in and simply clicks on the appropriate option within a patient's profile to document an intervention. In independent documentation systems, login time can be minimized through the use of saved passwords, biometric authentication, bookmarked links to the documentation Web site, and the use of login shortcuts that take the pharmacist to the desired documentation form. Some pharmacists will desire a portable documentation method, commonly performed on a personal digital assistant (PDA). Several of the approaches to faster login described also apply to PDA-based documentation (e.g., saved passwords and biometrics).

Once the pharmacist has logged into the documentation tool, it should be populated with any information pertinent to the documentation being performed. This information can include institution specific data such as clinical protocols, antibogram data, IV-to-PO (intravenous-to-oral) interchange guidelines, and the hospital's formulary. Patient-specific information can include the patient's location within the facility, admitting or primary physician, allergy history, current medication list, laboratory results, radiology reports, diagnoses, age, and weight. The availability of this information provides pharmacists with the information they need in a single location, creating efficiency by minimizing the need to access the information in a separate location. The availability of this information is greatly influenced by the type of documentation tool being used. Generally, commercial intervention tools (especially those that are modules of a larger information system) and tools developed by IS personnel are more likely to provide this type of information.

After pharmacists have reviewed the available information that allows them to make an informed decision regarding their patients' care, they then begin the documentation process. This is a critical point to impact speed in the documentation process. Here, the documentation tool should use quick-entry methods, such as drop down lists, check boxes, radio buttons, and other methods that allow documentation to occur with minimal (or no) typing. A well-designed documentation tool will allow a pharmacist to document an intervention without typing a single word. A well-designed tool will also provide the opportunity for free text notes to be entered into the documentation form, if desired, by the pharmacist. The key at this step is to ensure that as few clicks as possible are necessary to completely document an intervention while leaving the opportunity for free text entry, if desired.

An additional factor impacting documentation speed is using the minimum amount of data required to complete a documentation form. The documentation system administrator will have control over which fields are and are not required. The end-users of the documentation system should give their input to identify the minimum requirements for documentation. End-users will have valuable insight into the likelihood of their completing a documentation form based on the number of required fields they must enter for the form to be accepted. Balance should be sought to ensure that the form is not too long for the end-users but will, at the same time, capture enough usable data about each intervention documented.

Similarly, users should have the ability to document multiple occurrences of the same intervention at one time on an expedited version of the documentation form. Normally, this functionality only captures the number of a specific intervention and is not focused on other information, such as the patients involved, the medications involved, and the physicians involved.

Despite best efforts to ensure that the documentation form's length fits clinicians' workflow, there will be occasions when pharmacy practice does not allow time for documentation. For these situations, the documentation tool should allow pharmacists to save the form in its current state and complete it later. An additional useful feature would allow the person initiating documentation to save the form and "push" it to another user to complete (or sign off on) the form.

Step Four: Documentation

The most important factor contributing to the utility of your documentation system will be the ability for you to customize it to meet your needs. Customization is possible with documentation modules that are a part of your pharmacy management system and with commercial systems that exist external to your pharmacy management system. However, maximum customization is best found through documentation tools that you create, either with your IS personnel or through a commercially available database development application.

Customization of documentation systems focuses on tailoring the tool to your institution's needs. This customization allows the creation of a unique intervention table that lists all interventions specific to your institution. This customization should allow you to assign properties for each intervention, such as a consensus-based definition, time required, cost savings (hard and soft), and significance for each intervention. Other desirable, global customization includes the ability to create physician lists, intervention location lists, and medication lists specific to your institution.

One of the strengths of commercially available documentation systems can also be a limitation. Commercial documentation tools come with a prebuilt set of fields on the documentation form. As described, drop-down lists, radio buttons, and checkboxes can speed the documentation process. Additionally, these lists, buttons, and boxes can be customized to the institution's needs. However, this configuration creates the inability to change the actual name or descriptor of the field.

Most commercial documentation tools do not provide the ability to change field names. In the event that a documentation form does not contain a field needed by a specific institution, most commercial documentation systems do not give the institution the ability to change field names. This is a critical customization feature that can impact the utility of a documentation tool. Obviously, documentation systems developed in-house or through the use of database development tools will not suffer from this limitation. Recent conversations with documentation system vendors have indicated that they are aware of this need and are taking steps to address it.

Documentation form fields are also important for another reason related to customization. The need for a variety of user roles was defined earlier. Ideally, a documentation system will allow the administrator to specify which fields show for which user roles. This level of functionality provides true customization that allows the form to be tailored to a specific user group.

Customization for documenting interventions is important. An additional topic not related to customization but important to the documentation process is the ability to limit access to the documentation form. Whether documentation occurs on a PDA, an application housed on an institutional server, or a Web-based application, the documentation system should have an automatic lockout feature that logs the user out of the documentation form after a specified time period of inactivity. Obviously, this feature will prevent unauthorized access to patient information and documentation under someone else's profile.

Step Five: Reporting

From a pharmacy director's point of view, the reporting capabilities of a documentation system may be the most important feature. The ability to create informative reports that detail pharmacists' pharmaceutical care activities is critical in providing the director with quantitative data to support justification for personnel and resources. Identification and definition of reporting needs should occur before system implementation. This step allows the initial setup to be performed with full knowledge of the desired outcomes (i.e., data to report), which can potentially impact the intervention table and even documentation itself. For example, a pharmacy staff that has been performing IV-to-PO conversions for several years may elect to capture only raw totals of this class of interventions. In light of this, IV-to-PO conversion documentation would occur on the "expedited" form that focuses only on raw numbers. Other interventions that require more time and effort would be captured on the full documentation form because the director desires more data to present to the C-suite.

When considering reporting in general, as with the documentation process, "customization" is the key word. The reporting function should allow authorized users the ability to create reports that examine the specific fields and time frame desired. Users should be able to save report formats for reuse, and administrators should be able to create global reports that all users (or a set of users) can access and run by simply selecting the time frame desired. Additionally, users should be able to schedule reports to automatically run at predetermined intervals, capturing a certain timeframe of data, and send the results to a specified e-mail address. All reports should be created in a standardized format for export to a spreadsheet or database application for analysis.

Some institutions may find value in benchmarking their intervention activities with peer institutions. The utility and application of this capability has yet to be acknowledged in the literature, but applications of benchmarking are growing in popularity in other domains of health care. Indeed, the federal government's push for "transparency" across hospitals and providers in terms of costs and outcomes is closely related to benchmarking. Any pharmacy department pursuing benchmarking for intervention activities should ensure that peer institutions are comparable in terms of facility type (community hospital versus tertiary care teaching hospital), staffing models, clinical services provided, patient population served, and a host of other characteristics that impact the pharmacy's ability to perform interventions.

Other Considerations

Much of this discussion focused on steps that should be taken to maximize documentation by clinicians. In conversations with our community pharmacy colleagues regarding patient adherence to medication regimens, we often discuss the "best" reminder method for patients. Is the best method an e-mail, phone call, postcard, or something else? We believe the best method is the method that the patient prefers. Similarly, when creating a documentation system, the "best" method for documenting is the method the clinician prefers. Therefore, documentation systems should be designed to operate on any device a pharmacist would use. This device may be a standard desktop computer, a laptop computer, a tablet personal computer ([PC]slate or convertible), a PDA, an ultra mobile PC, or some device not invented yet. The take-home message is to select or design a documentation tool that is browser based and adaptable to small screens as well as large screens.

Two other considerations worth mentioning are well known to pharmacists. The documentation system's cost must not be prohibitive. While pharmacy department budgets continue to grow, the vast majority of budget allocations are for medications and personnel. The "out the door" cost of a commercial system should be carefully compared with the cost of an internally developed system with special attention given to the features described earlier. Ultimately, the decision of which system to implement will be driven by cost versus function. And when considering costs, initial and long-term technical support must be included in the decision process.

An emerging consideration is the importance of an online community of users. The Internet is rapidly transforming into the Web 2.0 model, which is characterized by online interaction and collaboration by individuals with common interests. This type of networking allows sharing of both failures and successes with intervention documentation. Much like the Pearls sessions at the Midyear Clinical Meeting, we find that some of our greatest lessons learned can be taught to us by our colleagues. Does your intervention documentation system vendor have an online community for collaboration? If you elect to create your own documentation system, what forum will you use to share your experiences with your colleagues? These questions should be carefully considered.

Conclusion

Pharmacy has progressed considerably from a focus on a drug product to a focus on patient outcomes and the pharmacist's responsibility for those outcomes. This transformation began with the clinical pharmacy movement and continues today under the pharmaceutical care model of practice. The literature is overflowing with examples of pharmacists' impact on patient care. The literature also describes different approaches to documentation of pharmacists' interventions on behalf of their patients. In conclusion, intervention documentation can be optimized by focusing on efficiency, user management, the documentation process, and reporting.

References

1. Francke GN. Evolvement of clinical pharmacy. *Drug Intell Clin Pharm* 1969;3:348-354.
2. Higby GJ. From compounding to caring: an abridged history of American pharmacy. In: Penna RP, ed. *Pharmaceutical Care* (2nd ed.). Bethesda, MD: American Society of Health-System Pharmacists; 2003.
3. McLeod DC. Clinical pharmacy: the past, present and future. *Am J Hosp Pharm* 1976;33:29-38.
4. Barker K. The future role of the hospital pharmacist in drug distribution systems. *Am J Hosp Pharm* 1967;24:220-227.
5. Hepler CD, Strand LM. Opportunities and responsibilities in pharmaceutical care. *Am J Hosp Pharm* 1990;47(3):533-543.
6. Penna RP. Pharmaceutical care: pharmacy's mission for the 1990s. *Am J Hosp Pharm* 1990;47(3):543-549.
7. Felkey BG, Fox BI. Informatics: the integration of technology into pharmaceutical care. In Penna RP, ed. *Pharmaceutical Care* (2nd ed.). Bethesda, MD: American Society of Health-System Pharmacists; 2003.
8. Brown G. Assessing the clinical impact of pharmacists' interventions. *Am J Hosp Pharm* 1991;48:2644-2647.
9. Hatoum HT, Hutchinson RA, Elliott LR, et al. Physicians' review of significant interventions by clinical pharmacists in inpatient care. *Drug Intell Clin Pharm* 1988;22:980-982.
10. Hatoum HT, Catizone C, Hutchinson RA, et al. An eleven-year review of the pharmacy literature: documentation of the value and acceptance of clinical pharmacy. *Drug Intell Clin Pharm* 1986;20:33-48.
11. Simonian AI. Documenting pharmacist interventions on an intranet. *Am J Health Syst Pharm* 2003;60:151-155.

The Catcher in the Rye: Learning from Community Pharmacists' Interventions on Electronic Prescriptions

Terri L. Warholak

Michael T. Rupp

Background and Introduction

In *The Catcher in the Rye* by J.D. Salinger, Holden Caulfield states that he wants to grow up to be the "Catcher in the Rye." That is, he wants to be the person who saves children from an event that he perceives as negative.[1] Pharmacists are, in a sense, the "catchers" of the United States healthcare team. In much the same way as Holden intends to catch children before a negative event occurs, pharmacists catch and intervene in medication therapy problems in order to prevent negative events from happening to their patients. As the "catcher" for the healthcare team, the pharmacist has a large responsibility in the implementation of electronic prescribing (e-prescribing) technology. Pharmacists must identify typical problems with drug therapy in addition to "catching" problems with the e-prescribing technology itself.

This analysis was conducted as part of a federally funded national pilot to evaluate e-prescribing in the community practice setting. One of the objectives of the project was to measure the incidence and nature of prescribing errors on e-prescriptions that resulted in active intervention by dispensing community pharmacists to correct or resolve.

Methods

A panel of participating community pharmacists reported their medication therapy interventions (MTIs) using either a standardized paper documentation form or an Internet-based tool created specifically for this project. The MTI documentation tools were designed to be compatible with the National Alliance of State Pharmacy Associations' (NASPA) Pharmacy Quality Commitment continuous quality improvement program peer review audit tools.

The authors declare no conflicts of interest regarding products or services discussed in this manuscript. This project was supported by grant number 1 U18 HS016394 from the Agency for Healthcare Research and Quality. Portions of this research were presented at the American Society of Health Systems Pharmacists Annual Meeting, Anaheim, CA, December 6, 2006.

NASPA's Pharmacy Quality Commitment (PQC) program is intended to be used by community pharmacies for internal quality improvement purposes. The peer review audit form was developed to assist community pharmacists to document quality related events in their practice such as dispensing-related errors that are identified before the medication leaves the pharmacy. When a quality-related event is discovered, pharmacists using the PQC program can elect to record the event immediately using PQC's Internet portal or note the event initially using a paper documentation form and transcribe the information into the Web-based tool at a later time. The Web-based tool, which is supported by a suite of analytical routines that produce graphic trends of the data, is designed to help pharmacists focus their quality improvement activities.

The authors decided to create a new form (both paper-based and Web tools) for this investigation because it was felt that the creation of such a tool would help pharmacists document therapy problems that originate in the prescribing phase of the medication process. In order to do so, the peer review tools were edited to include this shifted focus, and the resulting MTI reporting form is designed to allow pharmacists to quickly record their medication-related interventions. For example, if a pharmacist recognizes that the dose of a new e-prescription for amoxicillin is too high for a pediatric patient's weight (as listed in the patient profile), he or she may verify the child's weight with the parent and call the prescriber to change the dose. Such an intervention may take the pharmacist 6 minutes to perform and would be documented on the paper documentation form, as illustrated in Figure 11.1.

It is worth noting that, for this study, the tool focused on problems identified with e-prescriptions only. However, as can be seen in Figure 11.1 the tools can also be used to collect intervention data on all prescriptions regardless of transmission mode. A training excerpt for the online data collection tool appears in Appendix A.

Results

Data were reported from 68 participating chain pharmacies in five states during 312 work shifts between July, 2006 and September, 2006. During the study pharmacists reviewed 2,690 e-prescription orders (new, 83.0%; refill, 17.0%) and intervened 102 times for an intervention rate of 3.8%. The rate at which pharmacists identified problems on new e-prescriptions was found to be nearly twice that of refills (4.1% and 2.2%, respectively). The most common reason for pharmacists' interventions on e-prescriptions was to supplement omitted information (31.9%), especially missing directions. Dosing errors were also quite common (17.7%). The most common responses by pharmacists to e-prescription problems were to contact the prescriber (64.1%), consult the patient's profile or medication history (12.8%), and interview the patient or the patient's representative (9.4%). In most cases (56%), the e-prescription order was changed and the prescription was ultimately dispensed. In 15% of cases the e-prescription order was dispensed as written, following clarification by the prescriber. In 10% of cases the prescription was not dispensed. An additional 12% of prescription issues remained unresolved. A comprehensive report and discussion of the results of this analysis have been reported elsewhere.[2]

Discussion and Lessons Learned

Pharmacists who participated in this study were provided with both the paper-based and Web-based data collection tools. However, only one pharmacist opted to use the Web-based

Confidential

PLEASE PRINT   PLEASE PRINT

On the date shown I conducted the following interventions

to correct or resolve medication-related problems that were

identified from prescriptions that were sent electronically:

Zip code of pharmacy: _________________

Reporting Pharmacist (a four digit identifier known only to you) _________________

Day (circle one): M T W TH F SAT SUN   Date: _________________

Total e-Rxs I Reviewed/approved on this date: New: _________________   Refill: _________________

e-Rx Type (New, Refill, or Transfer)	Drug(s) Involved Medication: Name/NDC #	Drug(s) Involved Secondary or Conflicting Medication: Name/NDC #	Medication Therapy Intervention (MTI)					
			Rx Source (e-Rx)	How was the pharmacist alerted to the problem?	Reason(s) for Inter-vention (All that apply)	Pharmacist Actions (All that apply)	Results (All that apply)	Time Spent on Intervention (minutes)	Comments
N	Amoxicillin		e	4	C	1,2	B	6	Dose was too high for patient's weight.
			e						
			e						
			e						

Reason(s), cont.   **Pharmacist Actions:**   **Results:**

[1] PBM / Payer alert
[2] Physician notification
[3] Patient notification
[4] Pharmacist identified
[5] Pharmacy Computer system
[6] Other (specify above)

Prescribing Problems
A = Inappropriate Drug/Indication
B = Incorrect Patient
C = Excessive Dose
D = Excessive Quantity/Duration
E = Insufficient Dose
F = Insufficient Quantity/ Duration
G = Inappropriate Dosage Form
H = Drug-Drug Interaction
I = Drug Allergy or Sensitivity
J = Drug-Disease Interaction

K = Missing Information

L = Illegible
M = Violates Legal Requirements
N = Non-Formulary Drug
O = Additional Drug Needed

Drug Use Problems
P = Side Effects or Toxicity
Q = Over-Utilization
R = Under-Utilization
S = Patient Concern or Question
T = Possible Fraud or Abuse

U = Other (specify above)

[1] Prescriber Consulted
[2] Patient or Representative Consulted
[3] Profile/Medication History Consulted
[4] Literature Search/Review
[5] Other (specify above)

A = Dispensed as Written
B = Dispensed with Different Dose
C = Dispensed with Different Directions
D = Dispensed with Different Dosage Form
E = Dispensed with Different Quantity
F = Dispensed with Different Drug
G = Rx Not Dispensed
H = Drug Discontinued
I = Patient Education /Counseling
J = Other (specify above)
3/10/06
©2005, National Alliance of State Pharmacy

Associations, LLC

Figure 11.1. Electronic prescription (e-Rx) medication therapy intervention (MTI) report.

approach, possibly because many of the chain pharmacies in this study do not provide open Internet access to pharmacists and staff. In addition, several pharmacists mentioned that it was easier and quicker to incorporate the paper-based form into their workflow.

Most commonly, the reason for pharmacist intervention on e-prescriptions was due to necessary information that was omitted by the prescriber. To avoid such omissions, mechanisms should be implemented by physician e-prescribing applications and network switches to ensure that e-prescriptions are complete and contain all information required for legal and safe processing and dispensing. Failure to do so decreases medication safety as well as pharmacist and prescriber efficiency.

Dose problems were also frequently identified by pharmacists. Such problems indicate that the clinical decision support systems on the prescriber-side software are imperfect or not properly used. To ensure correct dosing, prescribers should make sure to enable and use e-prescribing decision support, and software vendors should work with clinical decision support functionality creators to improve these systems. When developing decision-support systems for e-prescribing, take special care and time in developing dosing error–prevention algorithms.

While e-prescribing appears to have virtually eliminated some traditional sources of medication errors (e.g., handwriting interpretation errors), it appears to have created new ones. For example, wrong drug errors were documented during this study. This was thought to be the byproduct of selecting the incorrect medication from a drop-down menu when using an e-prescribing program. It was the opinion of many pharmacy staff that persons other than the prescriber were actually generating some of the prescription orders and, in some cases, prescribers were not reviewing them before they were transmitted. Therefore, to achieve optimal patient safety gains, physicians should either perform their own e-prescription data entry or carefully review e-prescriptions entered by support staff before allowing them to be transmitted to the pharmacy. E-prescribing system safeguards and decision support should be developed to more closely scrutinize new prescriptions to prevent these errors. Because this is an extremely disturbing trend, the diagnosis should accompany every e-prescription as it is transmitted to the pharmacy. There is evidence to support that doing so will enable pharmacists to better identify these drop-down menu and wrong drug errors.[3]

Technology may decrease the incidence of certain types of medication errors while creating new opportunities for others. The results of this study support the need to monitor new technologies like e-prescribing for unexpected and unintended effects, including patient safety threats, negative impact on provider workflow, negative effects of pharmacy workflow, and cost. Information on e-prescribing problems can be used to create best practice recommendations and to make recommendations for technological improvements. By continuing to document problems with new technologies, such as e-prescribing, pharmacists can play an integral role in iteratively improving the implementation of technological innovations so that they may eventually product the benefits promised. Because doing so takes time, pharmacists should be paid for these services.

Conclusion

As currently implemented, e-prescribing technology still allows some traditional types of prescribing errors to occur and has given rise to new ones. On balance, it is hoped that patients are safer using e-prescribing technology. At the same time, it seems clear that pharmacists, as the "catchers" of the health care team, can play a major role in identifying problems with e-prescribing technology. With consistent reporting and subsequent iterative technological improvements, e-prescribing may eventually produce the safety and efficiency benefits promised.

Appendix A

How to Enter Medication Therapy Intervention Data Online

When returning to the site after registering, access the Pharmacy Quality Commitment website at "http://www.pqc.net/intervention" on your web browser. Click on the Medication Therapy Intervention (MTI) link found on the bottom of the menu on the left-hand side of the screen. This action will bring you to the registration site (see below). Because you are already registered, go to Registered Pharmacist Login and enter your username and password to log in.

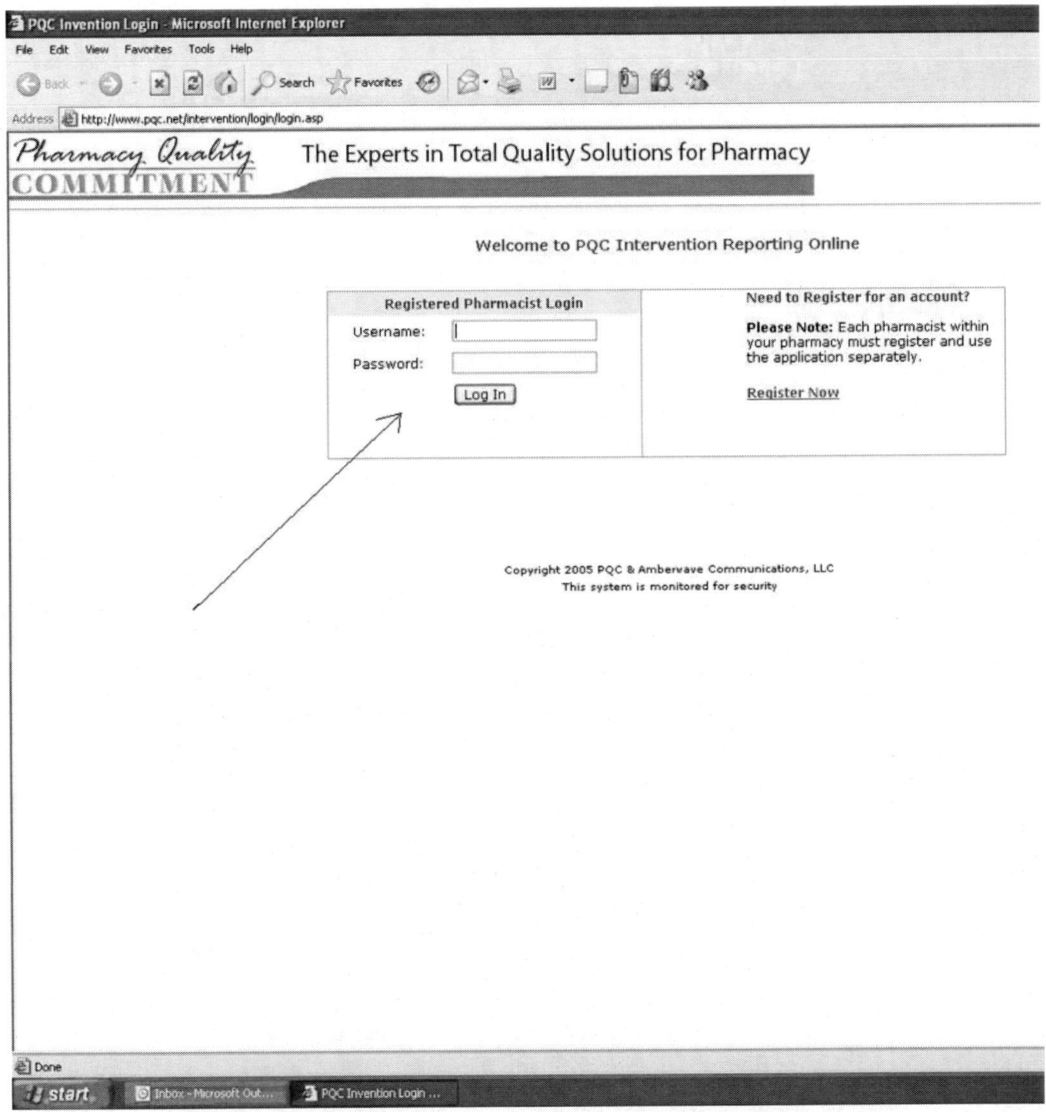

Figure 11.1. Pharmacy Quality Commitment registered pharmacist login.

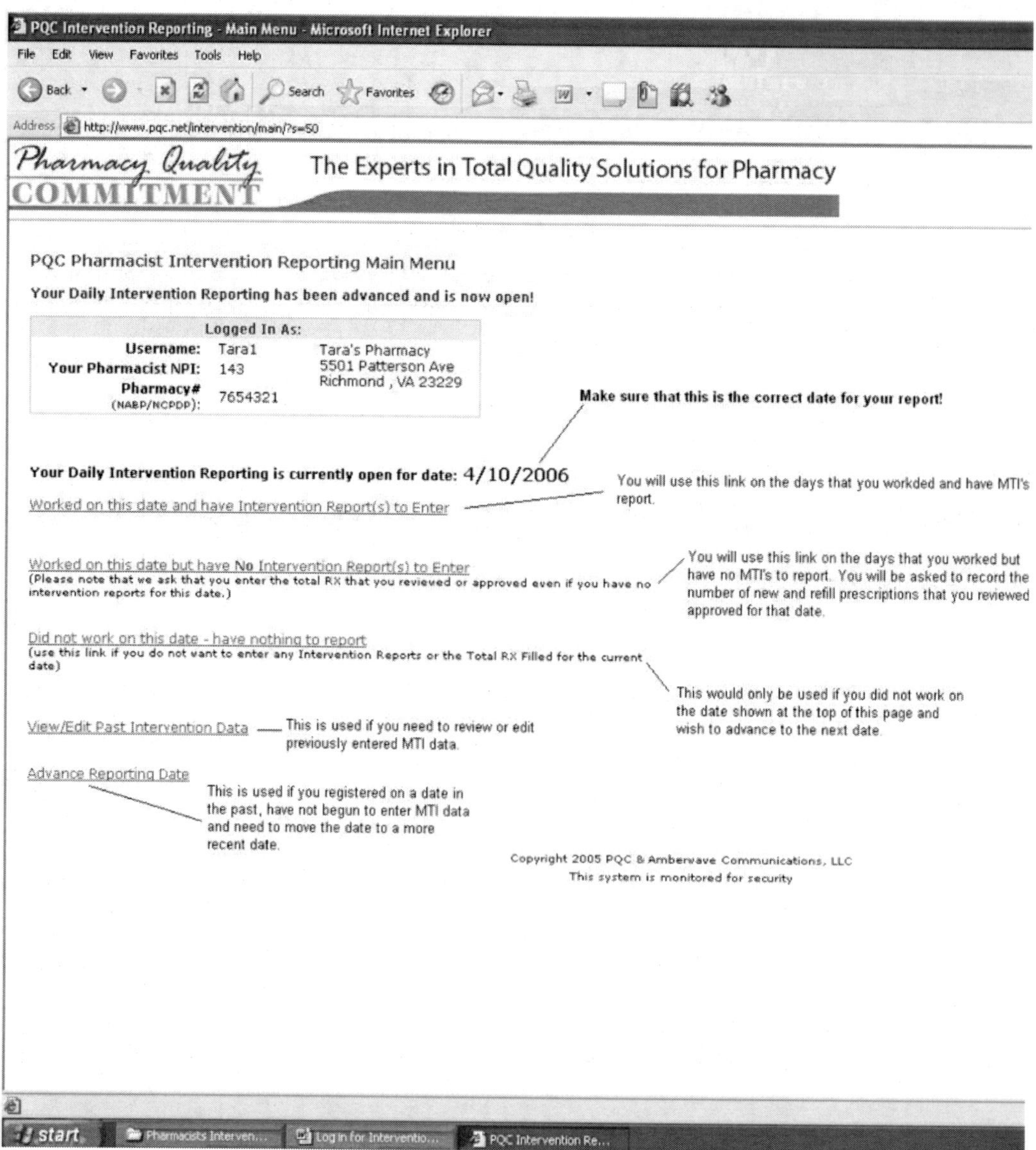

Figure 11.2. Pharmacy Quality Commitment pharmacist intervention reporting main menu.

Click on "Enter Intervention Reports" to enter your daily reports. Your screen will look like this:

This step will bring you to the last MTI report that you filled out—the date shown will be the last date that you entered an intervention report. Please check the date on the top of the report and make sure that it matches with the date of the MTI paper report that you are entering. Instructions on the online screen will help you if you need to enter data for a different day than shown, or if you have no MTI to report. This is the screen you will see during the day

Pharmacy Quality COMMITMENT — The Experts in Total Quality Solutions for Pharmacy

Main Menu | Log Out

Medication Therapy Intervention (MTI) Report

Entering an Intervention report for Date: 7/25/2006

Note: Please make sure that the date on your MTI reporting sheet corresponds with this date. A report should be entered for every day. If you did not work on this date, return to the main menu and click the 'Did not work on this date - have nothing to report' link. If you did work on this day but have no intervention reports to enter on this date, return to the main menu and click on the 'Worked on this date but have No Intervention Report(s) to Enter' link. If you did work on this day, and have interventions to report, find the MTI reporting sheet for this day and proceed to report.

Username: thebestpharmacy
Zip Code: 22222

Rx Type: **Rx Source:**

Drugs Involved

	Medication	Conflicting Medication
Name:		
NDC#:		

How was the pharmacist alerted to the problem?
    If other enter here:

Reason(s) for Intervention:
(check all that apply)

- ☐ Inappropriate Drug / Indication
- ☐ Incorrect Patient
- ☐ Excessive Dose
- ☐ Excessive Quantity/Duration
- ☐ Insufficient Dose
- ☐ Insufficient Quantity/ Duration
- ☐ Inappropriate Dosage Form
- ☐ Drug-Drug Interaction
- ☐ Illegible
- ☐ Violates Legal Requirements
- ☐ Non-Formulary Drug
- ☐ Additional Drug Needed
- ☐ Side Effects or Toxicity
- ☐ Over-Utilization
- ☐ Under-Utilization
- ☐ Patient Concern or Question

Figure 11.3. Medication therapy intervention report.

while you have the pharmacy open for business. You can enter your MTIs throughout the day as they occur, or enter the full shift's worth at the end of your shift.

Once you have finished your shift and are ready to finish up the day you will save your last report and chose the option to "store close for the current date." The final screen will ask you to record the total number of new and refill electronic prescriptions that you approved or reviewed on that date. After entering this information, click on "Submit." This step closes down your database for the day. You will then go through the same process as outlined for subsequent days of reporting.

References

1. Salinger JD. *The Catcher in the Rye.* Boston: Little, Brown and Company; 1945.

2. Warholak-Jackson T, Rupp MT. Analysis of community pharmacists' interventions on electronic prescription errors (in review).

3. Warholak-Juarez T, Rupp MT, Salazar TA, et al. The effect of patient information on pharmacists' drug use review decisions. *J Am Pharm Assoc* 2000;40:500-508.

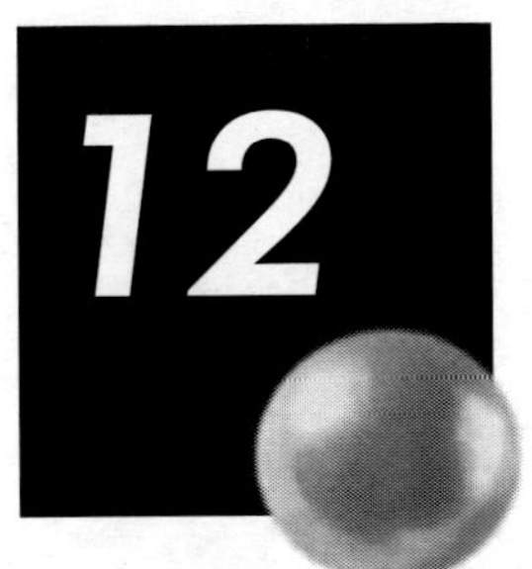

12 Online Pharmacy Services Resource Center: A Concept URL Bound to Love

Janet Jean Madsen

Background and Introduction

Turning my presentation at the 2006 Informatics Pearls session into this format was difficult because it was a guided tour comprised of 50 PowerPoint slides. The following overview gives you the flavor of the presentation and much of the content. If you wish to see the original presentation, it is available at the following address: http://www.ashp.org/s_ashp/docs/files/OnlinePharmSvcsResCtr.pdf. The information here includes updates since that presentation.

Readers can also go to Fairview's online pharmacy services resource center (www.formularyproductions.com/fps) and refer to it as you read this document. However, you will not be able to see behind the firewall. Many other hospitals that use the same vendor have all of their information accessible on the Intranet such as Wilson N. Jones Medical Center at http://www.formularyproductions.com/wnj.

Overview of Project

Overview of project

Home page—Left side

Measuring Usage

Formulary database: Information included on every drug page

Additional links which may be included on a drug page

Home page—center—a closer look at each blue bar

Home page—bottom area for news

Features and benefits of online pharmacy services resource center

Required skills to keep a good website

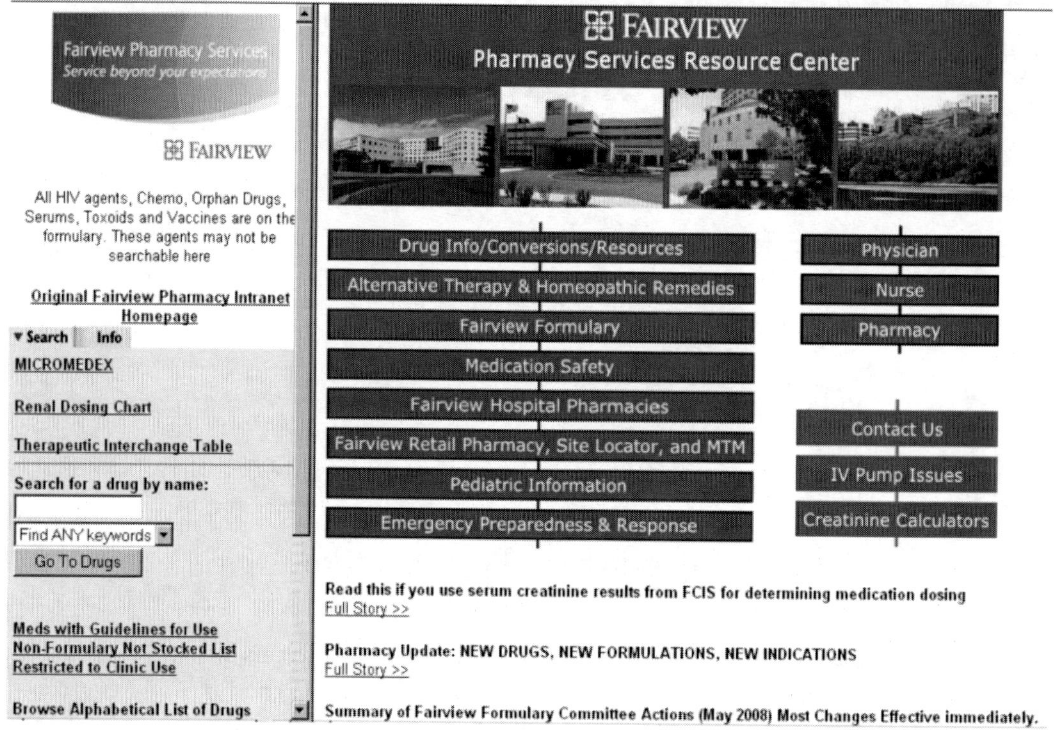

Figure 12.1. Fairview Pharmacy Services resource center.

Home Page

Here is the Fairview Pharmacy Services home page which is now accessible from a "quick link" on the Fairview Intranet. Starting at the upper left side of the page, users see:

- All HIV agents, chemotherapy, orphan drugs, serums, toxoids, and vaccines are on the formulary but may not be searchable here.
- They can still access the original pharmacy Intranet page, from before we had the added formulary capabilities from Formulary Productions.
- This is the place to click for quick access to:

1. Micromedex drug information
2. Renal dosing chart
3. Therapeutic interchange table.

- They can search for drugs by name.
- Fairview-specific information is provided, such as

1. Medications with guidelines for use

2. Non-formulary not stocked list

3. Restricted to use in clinics.

- An alphabetical list of drugs is provided.

Measuring Usage

There is a visit counter at the bottom left corner of the page. This site is being visited very regularly. We average over 6,000 visits per month.

302909 visits

Figure 12.2. Visit counter.

Formulary Database: Information Included on Every Drug Page

VANCOMYCIN
Meds with Guidelines for Use Click Here
BRAND NAMES: Lyphocin, Vancocin Hcl, Vancocin Hcl Pulvules
       CAPSULE: 125 MG; 250 MG
       POWDER FOR INJECTION: 500 MG
       SOLUTION (INJECTION): 500 MG, 1 GM, 5 GM, 10 GM VIALS
Comments See Guidelines for Use; Effective May 2008: Use oral solution in place of capsules (available at FPS Compounding Pharmacy)
Vancomycin Dosing Protocol
Pediatric Standardized Dosing
Antimicrobial Stewardship Policy
Kinetics Equations
Oral Vanco Soln Info

Recent Citations via Medline (PubMed)

Micromedex

E-Facts

Patient Information - CareNotes

Package Inserts

Figure 12.3. Formulary database: drug page.

Every drug page includes the following information:

- Generic name
- Brand names
- Forms and strengths available on formulary
- "Standard links," including:

1. Recent citations via Medline (PubMed)
2. Micromedex
3. E-Facts
4. Patient Information—Carenotes from Micromedex
5. Package Inserts

Additional Links That May Be Included on a Drug Page

Some drugs need more information. There are links to every Fairview policy, guideline, chart, and table that the drug is contained in. Please look again at the previous screenshot (see Fig. 12.3), where you can see that at the top you can click to review the guidelines for use for vancomycin.

FAMOTIDINE

BRAND NAMES: Pepcid

    SOLUTION (INJECTION): 10 MG PER ML
    SUSPENSION: 40 MG PER 5 ML
    TABLET: 10 MG CHEW; 20 MG GELCAP

Comments Non-formulary; Famotidine 20 mg oral is autosubbed with ranitidine 150 mg and famotidine 20 mg IV q12h changes to ranitidine 50 mg Q8H. Adjust for renal function and IV:PO interchange.

Pediatric Standardized Dosing

Renal Function Dosing Protocol

IV:PO Interchange

Recent Citations via Medline (PubMed)

Micromedex

E-Facts

Patient Information - CareNotes

Package Inserts

Figure 12.4. Non-formulary medication.

In the middle section, before the standard links, are links specific for vancomycin. All Food and Drug Administration (FDA) MedWatch alerts are linked in this area. If the medication searched for is a non-formulary medication, the formulary interchange, if one exists, is given (Fig. 12.4).

Home Page: A Closer Look

Now we will take a closer look at the 14 "buttons" in the center of the home page (see Fig. 12.1). Seven are divided by subject matter; three are divided by discipline (pharmacy, nurse, and physician); and the other "red" buttons are a contact button, IV pump issues, and creatinine clearance calculators.

Drug Information, Conversions, and Resources

Fairview's resources include the following (Fig. 12.5):

- Chemotherapy regimens and research protocols
- Do *not* put into *tube system* list
- Guide for IV hang time and tubing changes
- IV and chemotherapy information
- IV administration guide
- Standard drip concentrations
- Max concentrations
- Opioid conversion chart

Other resources include:

- Contraindications in pregnancy and lactation
- Cytochrome P-450 drug interactions
- Center for Disease Control immunization and vaccination information
- Organization and other healthcare links

Alternative Therapy and Homeopathic Remedies

- "All about Herbs" from Sloan Kettering
- Alternative therapy policy and procedure
- Homeopathic remedies policy and procedure

Fairview Formulary

- Formulary policy and procedure

- Formulary actions summary
- Drug class reviews
- Individual drug reviews
- Therapeutic interchange table

Medication Safety

- Instructions for reporting events, errors, and concerns
- Drugs with black box warnings
- Food-Drug interactions patient information
- Institute for Safe Medication Practices safety and hazard alerts
- The Joint Commission sentinel event alerts (medications)
- Some Fairview policies and procedures regarding safety

Fairview Hospital Pharmacies

- Phone numbers, addresses, and website links for the eight inpatient pharmacies
- System clinical expertise list
- Hospital residency program information

Fairview Retail Pharmacy and Medication Therapy Management

- ClearScript and National Pharmaceutical Stockpile Formulary
- Link to the Fairview retail website (www.fairviewrx.org)
- Insurance manual
- MTM information
- And more links

Pediatric Information

One bar contains links to all pediatric information originating from Fairview and other sources.

Physician

- Fairview resources (antibiograms, anti-infectives use guidelines, opioid conversions, etc.)
- Foreign languages aids
- Behavioral health resources
- Drug information links

Pharmacy (See Also Pediatric Bar)

Fairview Pharmacy System-Wide Policies and Procedures
System Pharmacy Policies and Procedures

Pyxis Troubleshooting
Pyxis Troubleshooting

FCIS Aids
WORx Information for FCIS
FCIS manual
FCIS Documentation Set-Up
FSH Acronyms
UMMC Acronyms

FV Dosing Cards

Adult Aminoglycoside Pocket Card
Adult Vancomycin Pocket Card

Warfarin Dosing Card
Warfarin Maintenance Dosing

System-wide PRN clarification list

Tools

MN Pharmacist CE Approval Form
Ideal Body Weight Calculator

BMI Calculator

Warfarin Dosing Website

Behavioral Health Resources

Consults Policy
    Includes PO:IV conversions for beta-blockers, benzodiazepines, ACEI, and Steroids
Cytochrome P-450 Interactions

Drugs causing Delirium

Drugs that need Hepatic Monitoring

Drugs in Pregnancy and Breastfeeding

Drugs in the Elderly Learning Module

Inappropriate Meds for the Elderly (Modified Beer's Criteria)

Feeding Tubes
    Med Administration via Feeding Tubes (UMMC P&P)
    A Guide to Drug Therapy for Enteral Feeding Tubes (Facts & Co)

Global RPh

Global RPh Calculators

Gluten Free Products

Grapefruit Interactions

Herbs, Botanicals and Other Products

Kinetics Equations

Kinetics Program
    PC must have MS Excel

Linezolid + Antidepressant
    Case Reports
    Progress Note

New Drugs Approved by the FDA by year

Figure 12.5. Fairview's online pharmacy resources.

Nurse

- Fairview resources (narcotic analgesic conversions, IV administration of medications guide, standard drip concentrations chart, and policy)
- Pyxis troubleshooting
- Foreign language aids
- Tools (clinical calculators, medication use with enteral feedings, etc.)

Pharmacy

- System-wide policies and procedures
- Pyxis troubleshooting
- Fairview clinical information systems information (computerized provider order entry)
- Fairview dosing cards
- An internally programmed Microsoft Excel kinetics program
- And many more links

Contact Us

Users can email the Web master (me) for quick responses to their questions, make suggestions, or report a broken link.

IV Pump Issues

One-stop reporting is provided for any and all IV pump problems.

Creatinine Calculators

Fairview's own process to take IDMS creatinine results and find traditional Cockcroft-Gault creatinine clearance values for drug dosing.

Home Page—Bottom Area for News

The news area on the bottom center of the homepage always has the most recent actions of the Formulary and Drug Use Committee and a Pharmacy Update with new drugs, formulations, and indications information and one link of local or national interest concerning safe administration of medication.

How to Create This Type of Online Pharmacy Resource Center

Fairview and many others used the services of Formulary Productions. Others, such as the

University of Kentucky, have created theirs in-house: http://www.hosp.uky.edu /pharmacy/formulary/default.html.

Features and Benefits of Online Pharmacy Services Resource Center

- One stop is provided for formulary information, policies and protocols, and drug information from many sources.
- Drugs are linked to the policies and protocols they are included in.
- Non-formulary therapeutic interchanges are readily available.
- Nurse, physician, and pharmacy-specific information is available at the touch of a button.
- Medication safety information is always available.
- Timely news items are easily accessible.
- Fast access to retail pharmacy information is provided.
- Fast access to therapeutic interchange table and renal dosing protocol is provided.
- It's available from any Fairview personal computer and to all others with portal access ("skeleton" to everyone).
- Information is downloadable to print and for personal digital assistants.
- Convenient and fast contact to Fairview Pharmacy Services is provided.
- The biggest benefit is that it reinforces systemization—Fairview Health Services comprises eight inpatient pharmacies in seven hospitals (the University of Minnesota Medical Center has two campuses on opposite banks of the Mississippi River), 32 primary care clinics, 43 special care clinics, and 26 retail pharmacies. This tool enables everyone to have fast access to identical information.

Required Skills to Keep a Good Website

1. Use Microsoft Windows.
2. Follow a cheat sheet.
3. Cut and paste.
4. Be motivated.
5. Be slightly obsessive-compulsive!

A website of this nature will always be a work in progress; as policies change, the FDA issues safety alerts and drugs are added to and removed from the formulary. It requires some time every month to keep this website updated. However, the benefit of having one place for everyone in our system to check for the latest medication safety information is invaluable.

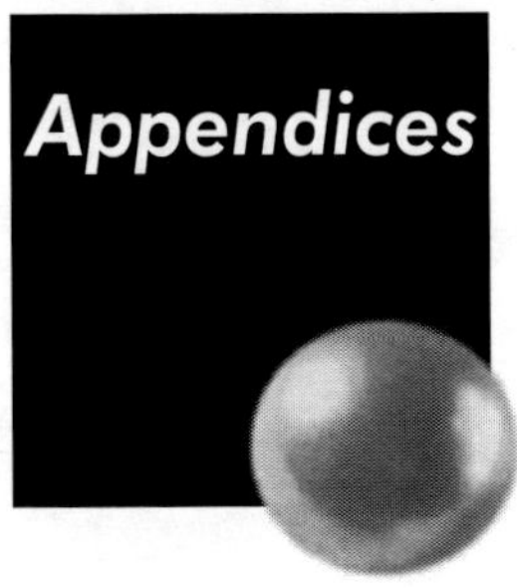

Appendices

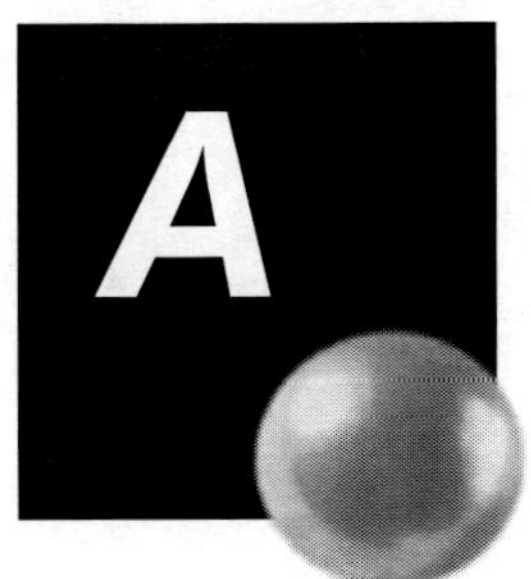

Appendix A: ASHP Statement on the Pharmacist's Role in Informatics

Position

The American Society of Health-System Pharmacists (ASHP) believes that pharmacists have the unique knowledge, expertise, and responsibility to assume a significant role in medical informatics. As governments and the health care community develop strategic plans for the widespread adoption of health information technology, pharmacists must use their knowledge of information systems and the medication-use process to improve patient care by ensuring that new technologies lead to safer and more effective medication use.

ASHP has long recognized pharmacy informatics as a unique subset of medical informatics that focuses on the use of information technology and drug information to optimize medication use. The purpose of this statement is to reaffirm the responsibilities of the pharmacist and the pharmacy informaticist in medical informatics.

Background

Medical informatics was first defined during the 1960s.[1] Since then, the term *informatics* has been redefined several times, reflecting the dynamic nature of the health care information technology environment. The National Library of Medicine defines medical informatics as the "field of information science concerned with the analysis, use and dissemination of medical data and information through the application of computers to various aspects of health care and medicine."[2] The central purpose of medical informatics is the dissemination of two core types of information: 1) patient-specific information created in the care of patients and 2) knowledge-based information, which includes the scientific literature of health care.[3] Most researchers consider medical informatics an interdisciplinary or heterogeneous field, made of individuals with diverse backgrounds and levels of training with an inconsistently defined set of skills.[4] The broad definition of medical informatics and the number of disciplines potentially involved present an opportunity for the growth of subspecialties within the field. One of these subspecialties is pharmacy informatics, which can be defined as the use and integration of data, information, knowledge, technology, and automation in the medication use process for the purpose of improving health outcomes. The potential for medical informatics to improve health outcomes has prompted the health care industry, large health care purchasers, and state and federal governments to undertake sweeping health information technology initiatives that commonly include the following applications[5]:

- Computerized prescriber-order-entry systems integrated with electronic health records (EHRs) and pharmacy information systems,

- Clinical decision-support tools that bring best-practice information and guidelines to clinicians at the time they need them and rule-based systems for monitoring, evaluating, responding, and reconciling medication-related events and information,

- Pharmacy information systems that allow electronic validation of medication orders in real time, provide the data flow needed to update both the medication administration record and order-driven medication dispensing systems, and support such operational activities as supply-chain management and revenue compliance,

- Automated dispensing cabinets and robotics integrated or interfaced with pharmacy information systems,

- Integrated medication administration management systems that enable the administration of bar-coded medications and use of "smart" infusion pumps, and

- Integrated medication surveillance applications for the reporting of medication incidents and adverse events.

Development of these applications requires organizations to reengineer existing medication-use processes by introducing additional technologies and applications to support the end-to-end management of medications across the continuum of care. The drive to create a seamless environment for realtime sharing of medication- and patient-related information across all levels of care has highlighted the importance of medical and pharmacy informatics in health care. Traditional pharmacy systems that focus on the transcribing, preparation, and distribution phases of the medication-use process are often considered the foundation, or hub, for communicating meaningful information outside the pharmacy domain. The creation of such systems requires a unique blend of medication management and technology-related skills and draws new attention to the need for pharmacy informaticists.

Federal Initiatives

Reports issued by the Institute of Medicine[6,7] and subsequent research validating the importance of technology in health care led the federal government's launch of two important health care technology initiatives. In summer 2004, the Department of Health and Human Services released a 10-year plan entitled *The Decade of Health Information Technology: Delivering Consumer-Centric and Information-Rich Health Care.*[8] The plan was specifically designed to transform the delivery of health care by building a new health information infrastructure that links health care records nationwide. The plan describes the pressing need to achieve "always-current, always-available electronic health records for Americans." These EHR systems would allow physicians and other health professionals to share valuable health care information at the point of care. The report identified four major goals[8]:

1. *Inform clinical practice.* Bring information tools to the point of care, especially by investing in EHR systems in physicians' offices and hospitals.

2. *Interconnect clinicians.* Build an interoperable health information infrastructure so that records follow the patient and clinicians have access to critical health care information when treatment decisions are being made.

3. *Personalize care.* Use health information technology to increase consumers' access to information and involvement in health care decisions.

4. *Improve population health.* Expand the capacity for monitoring public health, measuring quality of care, and accelerating implementation of research advances into medical practice.

The Centers for Medicare and Medicaid Services and the Department of Health and Human Services have published standards for an electronic prescription drug program under Title I of the Medicare Prescription Drug, Improvement, and Modernization Act of 2003 (MMA).[9] These standards are the first step in adopting final standards to address the MMA objectives of delivering cost-effective, efficient, safe, and high-quality patient care.

Electronic prescribing (e-prescribing) is the process of using a computer to enter, modify, review, and output or communicate prescriptions electronically to a patient's pharmacy.[10] E-prescribing with EHR systems further enhances the quality of care and patient safety by integrating the medication order into the overall process of medical care delivery.[8] Real-time access to patient information across the continuum of care and the provision of evidence-based clinical decision-support programs among stakeholders in the medication-use process offer opportunities to improve the quality of care, reduce errors, and improve workflow efficiency.

Pharmacists' Responsibilities

Pharmacists have unique, comprehensive knowledge about the safe and effective use of medications. More importantly, pharmacists understand core pharmacy operations and have developed expertise in end-to-end medication-use management, including communication with other information systems.[4] Pharmacists provide the expertise to effectively translate and seamlessly communicate the language of medication use across the continuum of care. They can interpret and implement requirements to ensure the safe and comprehensive communication of medication orders. An experienced pharmacist is skilled in the use of electronic medication-order-entry systems and has knowledge of human factor issues (e.g., interpretation of ambiguous clinical data) and the development of interfaces to disparate applications and systems.

Currently, there are many paths to becoming a pharmacy informaticist, with a growing number of training and residency programs focusing on this area. Although some pharmacy informaticists have formal academic or experiential training, the typical pharmacy informaticist is a pharmacist who has knowledge of computer systems, medication-use processes, safety issues, clinical management of medications, drug distribution, and administration and has developed extensive expertise in using technology to support these activities. Pharmacy informaticists are well suited to address the myriad issues involved with health care technology initiatives and provide leadership in the field of medical informatics. The pharmacy informaticist's responsibilities include active participation and leadership in all medical informatics activities that support medication use; education of pharmacy students, pharmacists, pharmacy technicians, health care colleagues, and administrators; and research on the core areas of medical informatics.

Participation. The active participation of pharmacists in all aspects of medical informatics that support the medication use process is imperative for safe and effective medication use. Such participation must be collaborative and comprehensive across the entire health care organization. It begins with system identification and vendor selection and includes identification of system requirements, as well as application design, development, implementation, and maintenance. Pharmacists must also be involved in the development and implementation of standards for medication-related vocabularies and terminologies to ensure safety and optimize deployment of activities related to clinical decision support.

Pharmacy informaticists are uniquely qualified to serve as liaisons between the pharmacy department and others involved in systems development, including vendors and other departments. The pharmacy informaticist's skills are needed to:

- Work closely with information systems and pharmacy staff to develop system programming requirements while understanding system capabilities and limitations,

- Develop and oversee databases related to medication management systems,

- Identify, suggest solutions to, and resolve system or application problems,

- Assess medication-use systems for vulnerabilities to medication errors and implement medication-error prevention strategies,

- Actively participate in the development, prioritization, and determination of core clinical decision-support systems, and

- Assist in mining, aggregating, analyzing, and interpreting data from clinical information systems to improve patient outcomes.

The participation of pharmacy informaticists in the enhancement of the knowledge management infrastructure related to clinical decision support will make it possible for more providers to access high-quality references, rules, and guidelines that are comprehensive, usable, actionable, and configurable. Enhancing the vocabulary and terminology infrastructure will make broadly applicable research on the effectiveness of specific clinical decision-support methods possible.[11] Depending on the size of the organization and its scope of medication services, one or more pharmacists assigned and responsible for pharmacy informatics may provide the best means for attaining the level of participation required for safe and effective information systems.

Leadership. Pharmacists are responsible for patient safety throughout the medication-use process and need to take a leadership role in medical informatics at all levels of health care to ensure that health information technology supports safe medication use. Pharmacy informaticists must use their skills to:

- Provide leadership to the institution's committees (e.g., practice, safety and quality, technology, pharmacy and therapeutics),

- Collaborate with other health care technology and clinical leaders to ensure that medication-related systems support interoperability and transportability of clinical information while maintaining patient safety and confidentiality,

- Attain key leadership roles within the health care technology industry, professional practice associations, and health care technology organizations, and

- Lead governmental and regulatory groups to sound conclusions regarding the use of technology in medication management, particularly as it relates to setting standards.

Education. Pharmacy informaticists need to develop a set of practical informatics competencies to manage medication-related data and information challenges across the continuum of health care.[12] Only a small percentage of U.S. pharmacy students currently receive the level of exposure to medical informatics needed to prepare for the dawning "decade of health information technology."[4] Pharmacy informaticists are responsible for providing strategic road maps for pharmacy educators that outline educational goals and objectives for training in medical informatics. Pharmacists actively involved in medical informatics within their own organizations are responsible for educating pharmacy staff and the institution's leadership about their role, particularly as it relates to using information technology to improve medication safety and quality of care. The education of leadership and staff must also include the inherent risks and negative aspects of implementing medication-use technologies. Their educational responsibilities include:

- Supporting the continued growth of ASHP-accredited informatics residency training programs by serving as informatics residency program directors and preceptors,

- Coordination and implementation of staff development programs and curricula in pharmacy departments designed to teach fundamental concepts related to technology and outline those areas of medical informatics in which pharmacists are critical to the development process (e.g., electronic prescribing and ordering, clinical decision support, drug administration), and

- Training pharmacy technicians in the use of medication-related computer systems and technology in an effort to develop roles for credentialed pharmacy technicians to support pharmacy informaticists and other pharmacy staff.

Research. Pharmacy informaticists are responsible for performing research involving the core issues of medical informatics. Such research includes the study of standards, terminology, usability, and demonstrated value involving the economics, safety, and quality of health information technology.[3] Research efforts should be focused on designing and conducting research to expand informatics knowledge and its use in supporting patient care. The pharmacy informaticist, through qualitative and quantitative research, can assist in determining the balance of clinical informatics and health care system reengineering needed to optimize the medication-use process and improve patient safety and outcomes.

Conclusion

Pharmacists have the unique knowledge, expertise, and responsibility to assume a significant role in medical informatics. As governments and the health care community develop strategic plans for the widespread adoption of health information technology, pharmacists must use their knowledge of information systems and the medication-use process to improve patient care by ensuring that new technologies lead to safer and more effective medication use.

References

1. Vanderbilt University Medical Center. What is biomedical informatics? www.mc.vanderbilt. edu/dbmi/informatics.html (accessed 2005 Dec 10).

2. National Library of Medicine. Collection development manual: medical informatics. www. nlm.nih.gov/tsd/acquisitions/cdm/subjects58.html (accessed 2005 Dec 10).

3. Hersh WR. Medical informatics: improving health care through information. *JAMA* 2002; 288:1955–8.

4. Flynn AJ. The current state of pharmacy informatics education in professional programs at US colleges of pharmacy. *Am J Pharm Educ* 2005; 69:490–4.

5. California HealthCare Foundation. Addressing medication errors in hospitals: a framework for developing a plan. www.chcf.org/documents/hospitals/addressingmederrorsframework. pdf (accessed 2006 Feb 9).

6. Committee on Quality of Health Care in America. Crossing the quality chasm: a new health system for the 21st century. Washington, DC: National Academy Press; 2001.

7. Kohn LT, Corrigan JM, Donaldson MS, eds. To err is human: building a safer health system. Washington, DC: National Academy Press; 1999.

8. Thompson TG, Brailer DJ. The decade of health information technology: delivering consumer-centric and information-rich health care. Framework for strategic action. www.hhs. gov/healthit/documents/hitframework. pdf (accessed 2006 Mar 10).

9. Centers for Medicare and Medicaid Services. Medicare program. Electronic prescription drug program; voluntary Medicare prescription drug benefit. *Fed Regist* 2005; 70:67568–95.

10. eHealth Initiative. Executive summary—electronic prescribing: toward maximum value and rapid adoption. www.ehealthinitiative.org/initiatives/erx/document.aspx?Category= 249&Document=269 (accessed 2006 Mar 10).

11. Teich JM, Osheroff JA, Pifer EA et al. Clinical decision support in electronic prescribing: recommendations and an action plan. Report of the Joint Clinical Decision Support Workgroup. www.amia.org/mbrcenter/pubs/docs/cdswhitepaperforhhs-final2005-03-08.pdf (accessed 2006 Feb 9).

12. Balen RM, Miller P, Malyuk D et al. Medical informatics: pharmacists' needs and applications in clinical practice. *J Inform Pharmacother* 2000; 2:306–18.

Developed through the ASHP Section of Pharmacy Practice Managers and approved by the ASHP Board of Directors on March 28, 2006, and by the ASHP House of Delegates on June 27, 2006. Copyright © 2007, American Society of Health-System Pharmacists, Inc. All rights reserved.

Mark H. Siska, B.S. is gratefully acknowledged for leading the drafting of this statement. ASHP also gratefully acknowledges the following individuals for their participation in drafting this statement: Louis D. Barone, Pharm.D.; James L. Besier, B.S., M.S., Ph.D.; Toby Clark, M.S., FASHP; Kevin C. Marvin, B.S., M.S.; Scott R. McCreadie, Pharm.D., M.B.A.; Sandra H. Mitchell, M.S.I.S.; John C. Poikonen, Pharm.D.; Michael D. Schlesselman, Pharm.D.; Rita R. Shane, Pharm.D., FASHP; James G. Stevenson, Pharm.D., FASHP; Perry D. Taylor, Pharm.D.

ASHP also acknowledges the following organizations and individuals for reviewing drafts of this statement: American Medical Informatics Association (AMIA); Institute for Safe Medication Practices (ISMP);

David M. Angaran, M.S., FCCP, FASHP; David Archer, B.S. Pharm., John A. Armitstead, M.S., FASHP; Anne M. Bobb, B.S. Pharm.; Paul W. Bush, Pharm.D., M.B.A., FASHP; Neil M. Davis, M.S., Pharm.D., FASHP; Charles De la Torre, M.S.; Doina Dumitru, Pharm.D.; Steven H. Dzierba, M.S., FASHP; Allen J. Flynn, Pharm.D., CPHIMS, CHS; Brent I. Fox, Pharm.D., Ph.D.; Mark Frisse, M.D.; Tim S. Fuller, M.S., FASHP; Greg Gousse, M.S.; Carol Hope, Pharm.D., M.S.; Janet Kozakiewicz, M.S., Pharm.D.; David Kvancz, M.S., FASHP; Rosario (Russ) Lazzaro, M.S.; Matthew Levanda, M.B.A.; Stuart Levine, Pharm.D. (ISMP); Lynnae M. Mahaney, M.B.A., FASHP; Patrick M. Malone, Pharm.D, FASHP; Henry J. Mann, Pharm.D., FCCP, FCCM, FASHP; John Manzo, Pharm.D., FASHP; and Michael McGregory, Pharm.D.

The bibliographic citation for this document is as follows: American Society of Health-System Pharmacists. ASHP statement on the pharmacist's role in informatics. *Am J Health-Syst Pharm* 2007; 64:200–3.

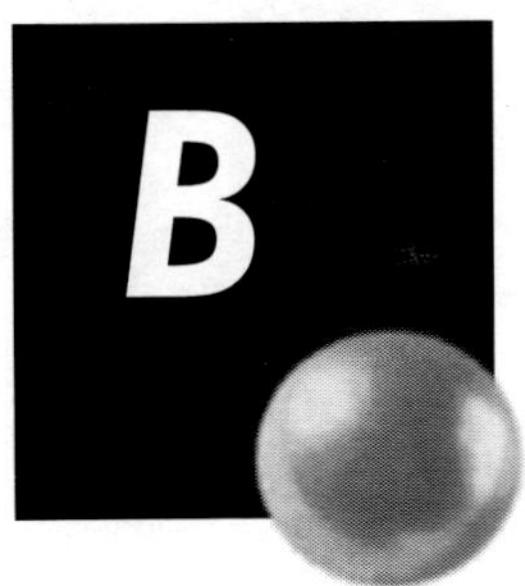

Appendix B: Pharmacy Informatics Specialty Residency/ Fellowship Programs

Please check http://www.ashp.org/informatics for the most current listing of programs.

Residency Information	University of Louisville HealthCare	University of Michigan	Sentara HealthCare
Location	Louisville, KY	Ann Arbor, Michigan	Norfolk, Virginia
Length of program	1-2 years	1 year (PGY2 only)	1 year
Informatics education	Project Management, Database, CPOE, Bedside Barcoding, Smart Pump Technology, Clinical Decision Support, EMAR, EHR, Wireless/Paperless Initiatives, Hardware/Software Systems Support, Teaching Opportunities	Prepare pharmacists to be leaders in informatics. Education will include technology concepts, project management, informatics research and education. Residents will be exposed to a variety of informatics topics and experiences.	Database design, maintenance, and reporting, CPOE/EMAR implementation, LAN/WAN technology, clinical decision support, interfaces, applications development, vendor relations, smart pump project, wireless technology initiative
Degree/ certification opportunity	None	None	None
Clinical responsibilities	At the discretion of the resident, informatics coordinator, and clinical preceptors	One weekend kinetic coverage monthly and one major, plus one minor, holiday	At the discretion of resident and clinical preceptors
Required clinics	None	None	General pharmacy practice residency or equivalent practical experience
Informatics projects	One primary plus multiple projects based on facility priorities	Projects vary depending on availability: two publishable papers	One major longitudinal project of publishable quality and multiple small projects throughout the year
Required rotations	Orientation, Project Management, End User Training and Support, Research/Study Support, Intelligent Clinical Decision Support Options, Database Design/Utilization/Mining. Infrastructure, Interface and HL7	Tailored to the resident's career goals	Project management, infrastructure, clinical documentation, clinical decision support, databases and applications, interfaces
Staffing	At the discretion of the resident, informatics coordinator, and clinical preceptors	Clinical staffing on required weekends only	At the discretion of resident and clinical preceptors
On-call pager responsibility	At the discretion of resident and clinical preceptors	None	Schedule varies
Residency directors and contact information	Amey C. Hugg, RPh, CPHIMS Pharmacy Informatics Coordinator 535 South Hancock Street Louisville, KY 40202 Phone: 562-3409 Email: ameyhu@ulh.org http://www.uoflhealthcare.org/Nurses PharmacistsandHealthProfessionals/ PharmacyDepartment/PGY2Informat icsSpecialtyResidency/tabid/534/Def ault.aspx	Scott McCreadie, PharmD, MBA, Strategic Projects Coordinator, University of Michigan Hospitals and Health Centers, UHB2D301, 1500 E. Medical Center Drive, Ann Arbor, MI 48109-0008 Phone: 734.615.2165 Email: srmc@umich.edu http://www.pharm.med.umich.edu/pu blic/residencies/informatics/	J. Miller Trimble, PharmD Pharmacy Informatics Specialty Residency Coordinator Director, Information Technology Sentara HealthCare 120 Corporate Boulevard Blding 400 Norfolk, VA 23502 Phone: 757.747.4607 Email: jmtrimbl@sentara.com http://www.sentara.com/Sentara/Emp loyment/Pharmacy/Residency/pharm acy_informatics.htm

Residency Information	University Health Care (Utah)	Brigham and Women's Hospital	St. Louis College of Pharmacy
Location	Salt Lake City, Utah	Boston, Massachusetts	St. Louis, Missouri
Length of program	1-2 years	2-year fellowship	1-year residency
Informatics education	Healthcare informatics with an emphasis on clinical applications, CPOE/e-MAR implementation, pharmacy automation, and private industry (TheraDoc).	Healthcare informatics, research techniques. Design, develop, test, implement, and create interventions that affect medication use. Measuring change related to an intervention will give the fellow the ability to conduct independent research	Clinical informatics (decision support, automated guideline monitor, CPOE and e-prescribing. Related research areas include acute care, managed care (PBM), and community pharmacy
Degree/ certification opportunity	Masters of Science in Medical Informatics or Masters in Public Health (Must apply for acceptance into the grad programs)	Master of Science or Master of Public Health from Harvard School of Public Health	Seeking ASHP accreditation (PGY2 Residency in Pharmacy Informatics)
Clinical responsibilities	Varies depending on clinical site, but similar to practice residents	Occasional teaching responsibilities at Massachusetts College of Pharmacy & Health Sciences-Boston	Variable clinical and teaching responsibilities in the area of pharmacovigilance
Required clinics	None	None	None.
Informatics projects	Varies depending on project availability, one major residency project required, project is presented at the Western States Residency Conference.	Minimum one, flexibility based on fellow's skills and interest	Multiple projects with at least one primary/longitudinal
Required rotations	Tailored to the resident	None	None
Staffing	Four 8-hour shifts per month	None, focus is on education, informatics, and outcomes research	None
On-call pager responsibility	None	None	Possible (daytime only)
Residency directors and contact information	Craig Herzog, RPh, MBA Director, Pharmacy Automation & Informatics University of Utah Hospitals and Clinics Department of Pharmacy Services 50 North Medical Drive Salt Lake City, UT 84132 Phone: 801.585.2188 email craig.herzog@hsc.utah.edu http://uuhsc.utah.edu/pharmacy/resident/clinical_informatics.html	Andrew C Seger, PharmD Senior Research Pharmacist Division of General Medicine & Primary Care Brigham & Women's Hospital 1620 Tremont street, 3rd floor One Brigham Circle Boston, MA 02120-1613 Phone: 617.732.5500 x33063 Email: aseger@partners.org http://www.brighamandwomens.org/primarycare/PDF/PharmacyFellowship.pdf	Terry Seaton, PharmD, FCCP, BCPS Professor Pharmacy Practice St. Louis College of Pharmacy 4588 Parkview Place St. Louis, MO 63110 Phone: 314.446.8524 Email: tseaton@stlcop.edu http://www.stlcop.edu/academics/residencydescription.asp?id=4

continued

Residency Information	Vanderbilt Medical Center	VA SAN DIEGO HEALTHCARE SYSTEM — A Division of VA Desert Pacific Healthcare Network	OREGON HEALTH & SCIENCE UNIVERSITY
Location	Nashville, TN	San Diego, CA	Portland, Oregon
Length of program	1 year (PGY-2 Preferred)	1 year	1 year (PGY2 only)
Informatics education	Information/Project Management, project lifecycle, technology infrastructure, integration/interface, implementation, CPOE, EMR, BCMA, pharmacy automation, vendor relations	Information/project management, data warehousing, internet-based applications, CPOE/Electronic Medical Record/BCMA maintenance, pharmacy automation	Information/project management, teaching, research, decision support, data warehousing, internet-based applications, training, drug information/drug policy, CPOE/EMR, evidence based medicine, vendor relations, pharmacy automation
Degree/certification opportunity	None	None	None
Clinical responsibilities	Mixed clinical and technical rotations at the discretion of the resident and preceptors	At the discretion of resident and clinical preceptors	Varies depending on clinical site, but similar to practice residents
Required clinics	Tailored to the resident	Tailored to the resident	None
Informatics projects	Multiple projects with at least one primary/longitudinal	Projects vary depending on availability	One 1-year long project and multiple smaller projects and , initiatives involving bar-coding, pharmacy automation and roles in the new OHSU health information system initiatives depending on availability
Required rotations	Tailored to the resident	No rotations, longitudinal residency	Medication safety, drug information/drug policy, experiences are longitudinal
Staffing	Every fourth weekend plus two hours each week, one holiday per year	Not required if resident has previous staffing experience as a general resident or as a pharmacist	Optional Schedule to be determined
On-call pager responsibility	Schedule varies	None	Schedule varies
Residency directors and contact information	Carly Feldott, PharmD Informatics Pharmacist & Program Director Vanderbilt University Medical Center 1211 Medical Center Drive . B101 VUH Nashville, TN 37232-7610 carly.feldott@vanderbilt.edu Office: 615.936.1992 http://www.mc.vanderbilt.edu/root/vumc.php?site=pharmacy&doc=6045	Daniel Boggie, PharmD Director, Pharmacy Data Applications (Daniel.Boggie@va.gov) or Jennifer Howard, Pharm.D. Director, Pharmaceutical Integrated Technologies (Jennifer.Howard2@va.gov) VA San Diego Healthcare System Pharmacy Service (119) 3350 La Jolla Village Dr. San Diego, CA 92161 Phone: (858) 552-8585 x 3026 Fax: (858) 552-7582	Mike Brownlee, MS, PharmD Informatics Program Director Assistant Director Oregon Health & Science University Hospitals and Clinics Department of Pharmacy Services, Mail code CR 9-4 3181 SW Sam Jackson Park Road Portland, OR 97239 Phone: 503.494.6054 Email: brownlem@ohsu.edu http://www.ohsu.edu/pharmacy/residency

continued

Residency Information	James A. Haley Veterans' Hospital & Clinics	PENNSTATE Milton S. Hershey Medical Center
Location	Tampa, FL	Hershey, Pennsylvania
Length of program	1 year	1 year (PGY-2 only)
Informatics education	Informatics program is based on core educational material from the American Medical Informatics Association and includes training in the VA's Hospital Information Systems. The program partners with industrial engineering departments of two universities to expose the resident to the more technical aspects of Informatics. Contact Program for more information.	Pharmacy information systems, & automation, CPOE, Clinical Decision Support, clinical documentation, process/workflow re-design, database, confidentiality, security, project management, system testing, user training, maintenance, and support. Strong multidisciplinary focus. Partnership with Cerner permits experience in commercial software design and implementation.
Degree/certification opportunity	None	None
Clinical responsibilities	At the discretion of the resident and preceptor.	At the discretion of the resident and preceptors
Required clinics	none	None
Informatics projects	One major project and various smaller projects involving automation and project management.	One major project, and multiple small projects throughout the year
Required rotations	No elective rotations are required but will be allowed with mutual consent of the resident and program director.	Clinical Workflow, Clinical Informatics, Medication Safety, Technology (Hershey and Cerner), Maintenance & Support, Decision Support, Project Management, Pharmacy Finance, Software Development
Staffing	Optional with dual appointment.	Required – Schedule will be determined
On-call pager responsibility	None	Required – schedule varies
Residency directors and contact information	Nicholas A Coblio, BSPharm, MSEM, PhD(abd), RPh James A. Haley Veterans Hospital Department of Pharmacy (119) 13000 Bruce B Downs Blvd Tampa, FL 33610 (813) 978-5804 nicholas.coblio@va.gov http://www.pharmacy-residency.com/index.htm	Dwayne J. Gallagher, Pharm.D. Pharmacy Informatics Specialist Penn State Milton S. Hershey Medical Center Academic Support Building 600 Centerview Drive (Mail Code A310) Hershey, PA 17033-0855 717-531-7296 (voice mail) 717-531-6162 (fax) email: dgallagher@psu.edu http://www.hmc.psu.edu/pharmacy/Residency/Informatics/informatics.html

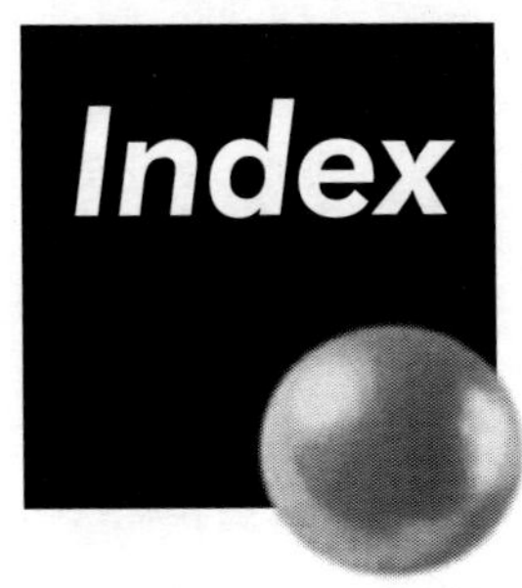

Index

Page numbers followed by "f" denote figures; those followed by "t" denote tables.

A

Adult learners, 9, 12

Adverse drug event form, 20, 20f

Andragogy, 8

Auburn University Harrison School of Pharmacy, 56–62

B

Barcode assisted medication administration, 27, 29, 43–45

Benchmarking, 61–62

C

Cancer registry, 48

Change model theory, 9–10

Children's National Medical Center, 33–36

Chronic fatigue syndrome, 48

Clinical pharmacy, 55

Communication, 34

Computer(s)

    downtime, 33–36

    tracking patient's personal supply of medication using, 38–42

Computerized provider order entry systems

    back-up for, 17

    benefits of, 15

    case study of, 7

    implementation of, 7, 15–17

    medication errors caused by, 15

    pharmacist's role in, 16–17

    prevalence of, 29

    success indicators for, 16

    training in, 7–12

Consultants, for information system, 3–4

D

Database

    development of, 57, 58t

    tracking patient's personal supply of medication using, 38–39

Department of Health and Human Services, 86

Diseases

    heritable predisposition to, 48–50

    high-risk pedigrees for, 50–51

Dispensing of medication using barcode technology, 27, 29, 43–45

Documentation of care

    description of, 55

    reasons for, 55–56, 56t

Documentation systems, for interventions

    access time considerations, 59

    account functions, 58

    benchmarking, 61–62

    building of, 56–58

    commercial, 57t, 60–61

    cost considerations, 62

    customization of, 60

    information, 59

    lockout features, 61

    online capabilities, 62

    purchasing of, 56–58

    reasons for, 55–56, 56t

    reminder methods for patients, 62

    reporting capabilities of, 61–62

    speed of, 59–60

    users, 58–59, 61

Downtime, 33–36

E

Electric data warehouse records, 49

Electric health record, 52

Electronic health records, 86–87

Electronic medical records, 29

Electronic prescriptions, 65–72

Electronic signatures, 22

Electronic systems, 25, 27

E-prescribing, 87

F

Fairview Pharmacy Services, 74–81

Federal initiatives, 86–87

Fellowship programs, 93–96

First-dose dispensing, 44–45

Forms, online, 19–23

G

Genealogical Index of Familiarity, 49–50

Genealogy data, 47–53

Genetic screening, 51

Greenville Memorial Hospital, 43–45

H

Health Alliance of Greater Cincinnati, 7–12

Healthcare system technology

    federal initiatives, 86–87

    training in, 7–12

Heritable predisposition to diseases, 48–50

High-risk pedigrees for diseases, 50–51

I

Influenza, 48

Information system

    organization support for, 1–2

    selection of, 1–6

Institute of Medicine, 25

Intervention documentation systems

    access time considerations, 59

    account functions, 58

    benchmarking, 61–62

    building of, 56–58

    commercial, 57t, 60–61

    cost considerations, 62

    customization of, 60

    information, 59

    lockout features, 61

    online capabilities, 62

    purchasing of, 56–58

    reasons for, 55–56, 56t

    reminder methods for patients, 62

    reporting capabilities of, 61–62

    speed of, 59–60

    users, 58–59, 61

L

Lawrence & Memorial Hospital, 1–6

Leadership, 88–89

Learning resources, 9

M

Medical informatics, 85, 88

Medicare Prescription Drug, Improvement, and Modernization Act, 87

Medication

    barcode technology for dispensing of, 27, 29, 43–45

    electronic prescribing of, 65–72

    patient's personal supply of, 37–42

    pharmacists' responsibilities, 87–89

Medication errors

    computerized provider order entry system-related, 15

    electronic systems for reducing, 25, 27

    e-prescribing, 68

    Institute of Medicine report on, 25

Medication management support systems, 29–30

Medication security envelopes, 40–41

Medication therapy interventions, 65–72, 69f

Medication-response phenotype, 51

Medication-use systems

    efforts to implement, 27, 29

    surveys regarding, 27, 29–30

Metabolomics, 51

Molecular genetics studies, 51

N

Non-formulary request form, 20

O

Online forms, 19–23

Online pharmacy services resource center
alternative therapies, 76
background, 73
benefits of, 81
drug information, conversions, and resources, 76
drug links, 76–77
features of, 81
formulary database, 75f
home page for, 74–75, 77–80
overview of, 73
usage monitoring, 75
Organization support for information system, 1–2
Oversight agencies for scientific studies, 52

P

Patient's personal supply of medication, 37–42
PDA, 22, 59
Pharmaceutical care, 55–56, 56t
Pharmacist
leadership role of, 88–89
responsibilities of, 87–89
Pharmacy informaticist, 87–89
Pharmacy informatics, 85–86
Pharmacy information management system, 29
Pharmacy information systems, 86
Pharmacy Quality Commitment program, 66, 69–70
Practice environment, 9

R

Relative risk, 49–50
Reminder methods for patients, 62
Reporting capabilities, of documentation systems, 61–62
Reports, 21
Request for information, 4
Request for proposal, 3
Research, 89
Residency programs, 93–96

S

Shore Memorial Hospital, 37–42

Staff development programs, 89

T

Training
computerized provider order entry system, 7–12
evaluation of, 11–12

U

Utah Population Database, 47–53